EMERGEN
of the
DIVINE
CHILD

healing the emotional body

EMERGENCE
of the
DIVINE
CHILD

healing the emotional body

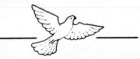

RICK PHILLIPS

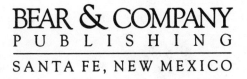

BEAR & COMPANY
PUBLISHING
SANTA FE, NEW MEXICO

Library of Congress Cataloging-in-Publication Data
Phillips, Rick.
    Emergence of the divine child / by Rick Phillips.
        p.   cm.
    ISBN 0-939680-67-X : $9.95
    1. Mind and body therapies.   2. Self.   I. Title.
RC489.M53E44   1990
615.8′ 52 — dc20   89-28386
                                                               CIP

Bear & Company
Santa Fe, NM 87504-2860

Cover & interior design: Kathleen Katz
Editing: Barbara Doern Drew
Typography: Buffalo Publications
Printed in the United States of America by R.R. Donnelley

9 8 7 6 5 4 3 2 1

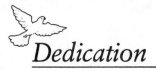

Dedication

To my wife, Paula:

Although I conquer all the earth,
Yet for me there is only one city.
In that city there is for me only one
    house;
And in that house, one room only;
And in that room, a bed.
And one woman sleeps there,
The shining joy and jewel of all my
    kingdom.

SANSKRIT

Table of Contents

Acknowledgments

I would like to symbolically thank Mother Earth for her nourishment and caring in my journey here and now. I would also like to thank:

Ann Phillips — for your difficult, but appropriate teachings as Mother for me in this lifetime. I love you!

Wendell Phillips — I wouldn't have done it any differently;

John Phillips — for just being a great brother;

John Oliver Phillips — a new soul for a new world;

Paula Kaufman — for your flexibility, simplicity, and obvious insights, but mostly for teaching me to love;

David Wright — for helping me face my denial;

Robert Wright — how about those Spurs?

Stephen Haines — for all your help, and especially your laughter;

Ralfee Finn — for new perspectives, namely "cat consciousness";

Lou Montgomery — for your inspiration for laughter & tears;

Dr. Kerry Tramontanas — for being such a good friend;

Julie Cooke — for being there when I needed you;

Peter and Melissa Evans — for introducing me to the whales;

Chris Griscom — for helping me get started;

Barbara Clow — just keep expanding my mind!;

Barbara Doern Drew — for your insightful editing & hard work;

Kathleen Katz — for your inner sight & outer expression;

Bear & Co. — for your outstanding job & constant support;

Shirley MacLaine — for the special times when you taught me dedication and commitment;

Devas everywhere — for everything; and lastly

our enlightened Chinese Chow deva, Moishe — for your unconditional love.

Introduction

BY LOU MONTGOMERY

I think a sign should greet us upon our arrival for earthly incarnation that reads: "Welcome back! School is now in session."

For myself, I try to hold the viewpoint that life's drama, with its outrageous Tarot-pack of players, the silly pratfalls as well as the tragedies, is simply curriculum, perfectly sequenced and designed to facilitate a single grand purpose: graduation, hopefully with honors. I find this viewpoint attractive for the simple reason that if I imagine myself enrolled in accelerated, upper-division courses such as Marriage 305, Forgiveness 603, or Neutrality 411, as opposed to merely surviving serial crises and getting scraped, bruised, and humiliated in the process, it is more interesting, far less depressing, and a hell of a lot funnier. Plus, I get credits. Why not?

As a great teacher of mine, Ron Hulnick, says, "Since most of our present and future reality is made up anyway, we may as well *win* in our own fantasy!" So, in my winning fantasy, I am successfully playing a myriad of roles, enacting a wide variety of outrageous scripts, and burning off tons of karma! Let's face it, it gets tediously boring to play the same victim role millennium after millennium and to insist on taking it so seriously. As my friend Errol Strider jokes, "When all else fails, take it personally."

So I choose to envision all of us as learners in the most prestigious university in the galaxy. And quite lucky we are to be enrolled here in Earth school even in these crucial times when tuition itself is costing us the very air we breathe and water we drink. Part of the ongoing curriculum seems to involve being conscious custodians of our fragile planetary home — maintaining an environment conducive to optimal learning. Despite the mounting evidence that we humans have become, as Joan Halifax has stated, the "pathogens" of Earth, and are at best remedial when it comes to learning from our past and at worst slavishly addicted to fouling our nest beyond repair, more and more of us have begun the fearsome task of cleaning up our inner environment, the "toxic waste dump" that has accumulated in our own emotional bodies. And fortunately we are blessed to have among us healers of insight, integrity, vision, and courage to assist in the cleanup.

Rick Phillips, one such healer, has over the past several years assisted immensely in the clearing of many people's emotional and mental baggage, including my own, and has become a close personal friend and treasured fellow accelerated learner. In *Emergence of the Divine Child*, he writes with exceptional clarity about the curriculum of the soul's sojourn during earthly incarnation, and provides us with refreshingly inspirational examples of transformation drawn from his life experience.

Many people know me by virtue of having seen me on some stage or another, and might view me as an audacious and energetic funny lady who writes and performs comedy about the not-so-funny topic of addiction recovery and societal and family dysfunction. Other people also know me as a teacher, for I have been privileged to work for the past seven years at a unique school in Santa Fe, NM — the Southwestern College — where masters-level students are trained in transformational counseling and creative expressive therapy. As an artist-healer, I am an outspoken and passionate lover of my work because it is fun, rewarding, and a constant surprise. I never know what or who I will create next! But this is recent history. I am also a recovering codependent and an adult child of alcoholics.

Not unlike Rick's story of his own family history, I lived most of my life, as an adult child of alcoholics, in trench warfare. I alternated between launching full-out assaults in order to protect a "front" of productive, acceptable normalcy, and then retreating, drained and exhausted, into an abyss of denial, distractions, and relationship addiction. For years, I maintained a virtual arsenal of projects, distractions, emotional soap operas, and, of course, an endless replacement of men, to cover up psychic and spiritual emptiness. The amazing thing is that I managed to immerse myself in a cozy bubbly-bath of New Age therapies and personal-growth seminars for more than fifteen years and still conveniently sidestep the fact that I was a deeply wounded codependent whose life was completely unmanageable. The tenacity of my denial alone has deemed it worthy of my admiration; for it has proved itself to be what Don Juan might call "a worthy opponent." In addition, I suppose I was ardently committed to what Pir Vilayat Khan calls "the spiritual bypass."

I began my recovery about four years ago, but, of course, had no idea that was what it was. I had just read Barbara Clow's account of her past-life regressions in *Eye of the Centaur,* and was planning to depart for Britain to make a documentary film about ancient sacred sites and geomancy. I, too, wanted to "tap into" my no-doubt sensational Celtic, Druidic, Arthurian epic lifetimes and write off the sessions as a "research" expense. Being a typical Santa Fe light-tripper, I simply phoned up The Light Institute, which was then still something of a local "best-kept secret," slipped through a crack in the normally backlogged schedule, and within days found myself lying on a table in Galisteo.

Rick Phillips was my facilitator — a charming, bright-eyed, sensitive man with a drawl. I bonded quickly with this fellow Texan who was not only adroit with acupuncture needles, but was, as it readily became apparent, profoundly safe and perceptive. What I was to experience in those first sessions was *not* the spiritual bypass. Nor was it the epic recall of my lives and times as a shape-shifter, high priestess, or galactic temple record-keeper. For certain there were some altered-consciousness bells and whistles, dimensional shifts, and visitations of beings who manifested to my High Self as everything from time-traveling, talking dragons to the Hindu fire god, Agni. (For all I knew, as addicted to drama as I was, my High Self was just keeping me entertained while something far more profound was taking place. The High Self will present material stored in the emotional body in whatever form grabs our attention to facilitate healing.) What transpired instead over the next four days was the release of deep emotional scars and imprints accumulated over lifetimes of confusion, abuse, self-neglect, and habitual, fixated, thinking and feeling patterns. All of these, like other addictions, had demanded higher and higher doses over time, while simultaneously increasing in their toxicity and harmful consequences.

My most deeply corded and painfully enmeshed relationship tie was with the personage who had manifested in this lifetime as my rage-aholic and alcoholic mother. At the time of my second session with Rick, my mother was lying bedridden in a coma, as she had been for weeks, emaciated and ravaged by chronic alcoholism, drug addiction, and cancer. In that session with Rick, lifetimes were flashed before me like a Rolodex. My High Self displayed what seemed to be every possible combination of relationship roles with my current mother as were conceivable, and ultimately took me back to an existence that I can only describe as "gaseous" — perhaps before I even began my human incarnations. At that point, the imprints fully let go at the cellular level. The vacuum thus created in my emotional body was lovingly replenished by a flood of indescribable light, joy, and ecstasy. Within hours of the completion of the session, my mother gently turned loose of her ravaged physical shell and passed over. From my point of view, our eons of mutual karmic abuse had lifted and resolved peacefully. Though she died hundreds of miles away, the heartfelt forgiveness and profound appreciation I felt for the incredible learnings she had facilitated throughout our stormy history must have eased her torment and assisted in her transition. An immeasurable gift was brought to me that day from Spirit. It was also to be the beginning of an intimate, trusting relationship between Rick and myself, for we have continued to work together periodically ever since.

The chapters that follow recount healings, perceptual shifts, and realizations no less dramatic or moving than my own. Also, the book is quite instructive as to how addictive emotional patterns shape our karmic destinies and act as a timely, illuminating bridge between the fields of recovery and past-life regression. Prepare yourself for an adventuresome learning experience. School is in session!

Lou Montgomery
Expressive therapist and performance artist
Chairperson of the Creative Expressive Therapy Department,
    Southwestern College
November, 1989

The Beginning

*A*ll is One. The Oneness is. The light is such a soft light, so intimate, a comfort. . . . It seems so omnipresent and yet so personal. I am here and yet I am everywhere; I am a soul and yet I am part of the whole. My vision is clear, and I can see my source, my purpose, and my path. The path has been long, and I have chosen many lifetimes to experience the meaning of life.

I am a witness to this awareness of unity, and yet I maintain an identity. I know I am part of the Oneness, yet I still have a spirit form that separates from the Oneness. I realize that this is my path: to bring this separation into completeness . . . a merging into unity. It is such a joy — intimate bliss — to be back in this feeling after the labors of my recent lifetimes, and I know it is time to understand what I have to resolve in my karmic history.

I look back at the progression of lifetimes. I see the growth, the evolution, of my consciousness, and I see the limitations, the unresolved attachments, of my emotional body. Yet I see the perfection of these attachments in my journey — how they are the opportunities for me to experience emotion, the juice of life; how we are all on this journey, yet each experience is a unique, individual journey. Everything happens in a perfect way. Nothing is without meaning. It is all synchronized in the cosmic flow . . . like the beautiful spiral nebulae, all flowing coherently on and on.

For this brief time between lifetimes I am outside the limitations of form, yet I remember the other viewpoint while in a body, of looking into the sky and seeing only the chaotic scattering of stars of the Milky Way Galaxy. Oh, how our point of view affects our perception of what we call "reality"! My reality of now being free of the body is so different from what was before and before and before. . . . What illusions we hold onto, but what a great teacher the experience can be.

I am now feeling the silent ecstacy of this expanded point of view. . . . Will it grow even more grand the next time I arrive on this transition platform? After my next life will it be even more contrasting? Can I know this while in a body? What choices can I make to know God permanently? Of course, this is my path . . . and I realize that path is glorious. For so long I felt the grip of the illusion of time always propelling me forward toward the "goal" . . . as if one day, after so much struggle, I would reach the "goal" and then I'd be happy; if I would work hard enough, or follow the Commandments long enough, or promise to be patient enough, one day I'd find it and I would be fulfilled. What an irony! It follows the great cosmic joke of what human life is about — cause and effect, the dance of yin and yang — but here on this spirit level, we know that the answer is *in the moment*, in the transcendent, in the recognition of the silent source within us. We don't have to do anything! Just *be*.

To be back in this spiritual dimension again also reminds me of all the divine souls that have traveled through so many lifetimes with me — playing the roles for me, so that I would be able to see from many different viewpoints. On Earth, it's like being an actor and playing on the stage — we keep choosing different roles, so as to be able to understand each particular reality, to experience the diverse ways of behavior, attitude, and emotion. Human life is rich in possibilities, yet each new choice is always appropriate for ourselves and our environments. Because the beauty of perfection is that other souls choose to relate to me as much as I do to them; this is synchronized so that we each receive what we need. No one is forced to play the part; we have spiritual free will, whether we choose the victim or the victimizer.

Being in the light again is like finishing the play and taking the mask off. The role having been completed, we have now come home to our Self. We can just be ourselves. But soon we choose another mask to wear to dramatize life one more time, to gain the treasured experience of being another actor. The question is, for how long do we keep putting on the mask? When do we know that we have accomplished our mission, our purpose? When do we learn the lessons of our experiences? When do we realize that we are not the mask and role with which we have been identified?

I feel I am close to really knowing the answers to these questions while I'm in the body. Everything is so clear here in the spiritual dimension, but there have been countless times on Earth when my vision was opaque to this knowledge.

It is really so simple. Silence is simple. Orderliness, by definition, is not chaotic or complex. Oneness knows no diversity, separation, or inhibition. Oneness just *is*, and all is One. Now I am coming back into a human body for the grand finale. . . . And now I'm born again.

One

Preparation for a New Birthing

In Earth are founded all the worlds.

RIG VEDA (6.5.2)

Following the thought
with the heart
He has reached knowledge
of the light.

RIG VEDA (3.26.8)

I was born with a purpose. My work today of helping people to find their inner guidance is the manifestation of that purpose. Of course, looking back at my life, I see how I started in denial, in conflict — how I set the stage with many obstacles and difficulties, but also with the tools to transform the conflict into growth, the obstacles into opportunities. This is the way of evolution on this planet.

Isn't it interesting how universal the theme of denial is! Everyone around me could see my problem, the emotional issue that had me in its grip, but I reacted by saying, "You're wrong

1

— it's not true." Looking honestly, without fear, without block-ing, was and continues to be a true challenge, one that we each must master.

I have picked two parents and a brother who have played the role of master teachers when it comes to my theme of denial. They were the mirrors that kept bringing me home to my karmic lessons. Every time I would say, "Can't you see what *your* problem is?" I would be giving myself an opportunity to look at myself. These three souls that I have chosen even had the incre-dible strength of love to play their roles in the extreme so I could get the point. My mother, "the alcoholic," who through her drinking destroyed her life, denied her brilliance and pushed away her loved ones. My father, "the alcoholic," who denied the downfall of his life, choosing not to see what was happening to him and around him, is now physically blind. The symbols of the alcoholic and the blind man are important because they represent the themes of, for my mother, "Let me continue the addiction of escaping and anesthetizing my life so as not to feel the pain of living"; and for my father, "If I don't *see* my life, maybe I won't be overwhelmed by it."

This scenario reminds me of the proverbial ostrich with its head in the sand. These are classic symbols of denial, which are created from past trauma and pain, and perpetuated by the fear that they will be repeated. Whether or not the trauma repeats, the fear of it is enough to make it a living reality within our awareness. The fear will manifest into expression when someone or something pushes the appropriate button to trigger our response. I have witnessed this repeatedly in my beloved, yet dysfunctional, family. I'm grateful now that I have the under-standing to thank my parents instead of blaming them for my upbringing.

My brother is the classic child of alcoholic parents, and like them, he is struggling with his blockages to intimacy and freedom of emotional expression, while holding all the old pain inside so that his physical body is slowly disintegrating under the pressure.

I have seen my contribution to my brother's struggles, and, sadly, it has taken years to change my old, habituated behaviors of anger, the need for power and self-doubt, and the need for approval that I projected on my brother. He felt the burden, and it pushed him into a defensive stance of insecurity and separation. It is interesting that when he was younger he had hearing problems and speech difficulties in interpersonal communication.

A child of alcoholic parents suffers through most of the typical alcoholic behaviors, but without the physiological effects of the alcohol. He or she picks up the energy of the alcoholism through the role modeling and the subconscious patterning of living in and around the emotional "field" that radiates and permeates the fabric of family relationships. The child may learn how to be unreliable or emotionally unavailable, to be angry and aggressive, or even to mirror the mood swings that he or she continually witnesses in the alcoholic parent. But the serious imprinting comes from watching how the parent deals with problems in life and the resulting disintegration of self-respect and self-confidence due to the overwhelming effect of self-judgment and guilt. The child has no model of normalcy or sense of what is "functional." Dysfunction is the norm and the template for future relationships. My brother and I experienced this behavior pattern intensely, and from my perspective, he was especially scarred from it.

Later in life, my brother found the beginnings of salvation from our grandparents, who became his role models, his "real" parents, who showed him stability. He could depend upon them; they were emotionally available. In the meantime, his animals became and still are today his outlet for love. Like many children of alcoholics, my brother directed his heart energy to the source that would never reject or disappoint him. He found that his animals could give unconditional love, whereas his family could not. His pets would not judge him, and would always be available. Only now, through a marriage to a loving and patient woman and the birth of a son, is his heart chakra opening to human relationships.

I remember my mother as the family philosopher. Growing up we spent hours talking about Aristotle, Plato, Eastern philosophy, religion, government, music, utopia. It kindled the spark of hope into a flame within me. As a young boy I remember writing school term papers about the search for utopia and utopian societies. In the sixties, I was happy to see people attempting to find or create an environment of peace and prosperity — coming to value the slogan "small is beautiful," treasuring the perfection of nature, and living in natural settings. We were trying to transform the Industrial and Technical Revolution into a balanced human/nature *consciousness* revolution. For a teenager in the sixties, the world was full of possibilities and new alternatives with a heart — the dream was being dreamed.

Somewhere things went awry. Our limitation was our lack of maturity — we had not yet learned the lessons we needed to bring our dreams to fruition. Our technologies of consciousness, such as meditation and other traditional forms of inner discovery, were overshadowed by the use of drugs and an inadequate connection to the "divine knowing" within us. We needed more time to prepare ourselves for the challenges — twenty years, to be precise. Now, here we are. We have grown, learned many valuable lessons since those chaotic times. We have matured. Of course, we still have a long way to go, but we have a foundation to build upon, and the New Age is dawning.

My parents were the philosophers, the scholars of life and living. My mother (feminine symbol) was the spokesperson and my father (masculine symbol) the manifestor. They had the knowing; they had studied how philosophies developed and collapsed. They could learn from the historical teachings. My parents were incredibly intelligent and had been given the intellectual and social resources to manifest their dreams, to create an enlightened life for themselves and their family — and to model that example to the world around them.

What happened? Their dreams did not manifest. Somehow their lives took another path, a different set of choices; somehow the world of ignorance overwhelmed them. My mother became the disillusioned philosopher, "the fatalist." She started drinking and smoking, and became numb to her dreams. She chose to destroy herself and say to the world, "It can't be done; there is nothing I can do!" My father became impotent, no longer able to manifest — the dream he shared with my mother had been denied. He began to drink and go blind, so he wouldn't see what could have been and, more importantly, what *was*. These are the parents I chose and the roles I chose for them to play. I played my part within the drama of life multidimensionally: within the dimension of my family, within the dimension of the society, and also on the level of my personal self.

Denial is due to a choice to close and lock the door to some aspect of life. This shutting down of a feeling creates an energy blockage within us. My parents mirrored this lesson of how our hopes and dreams can be annihilated by the fear of failure (which many times creates failure) and the choice to close down our feelings instead of taking the risk to confront what we attract to ourselves emotionally. By denying, we choose not to learn, and by not learning, we stagnate and feel stuck and defeated. When we realize that we can learn and grow from any experience, our ability to embrace life will be enhanced.

We may laughingly say that "ignorance is bliss" or "denial is bliss." This may be true temporarily. Eventually, however, ignorance and denial create the opposite effect. Maybe the degree of "hell" we have created on this planet is the impetus that is required for us to break free and create "heaven on earth" in a way that will not be forgotten easily. To an addict/alcoholic, vigilance is required in working "the recovery program" for the rest of this life. To a Jew, the Holocaust is never forgotten. Once we have opened the door of our denial, we must be careful not to close it again.

I was born with great potential, which I chose to manifest on the level of my physical body during my boyhood. By the time I was six years old, I had excelled in every sport. Between six and thirteen years of age, I never lost a swimming race, lead my baseball league in home runs, no-hitters . . . almost everything. I had a feeling that I could do anything, and nothing could stop me from fulfilling my desires.

As I grew older, I discovered I was no longer the best. I experienced defeat, a weakening of my self-confidence. I worked harder and harder, but there were always people who could defeat me, who expressed greater talent. The message became loud and clear: "You're no longer the champion." I didn't like that — I had been programmed that I would be appreciated only if I was on top. I worked still harder in training, until one day I collapsed in total physical exhaustion. The doctor said I had to quit or cut back. So I quit.

It was time to evaluate what was happening to me. I was seventeen. Somewhat typical of adolescent consciousness, I rejected athletics and joined the social crowd. Looking back, I think this time of craziness was when I started to express the emotional energies of guilt, fear, and vulnerability that I had repressed and controlled. As the feelings were triggered, I felt the terrible confusion of doubting all my previous accomplishments and my ability to deal with this new reality. The anger at myself seemed to be the most intense. I projected it onto everything around me, and as a result, I found myself feeling more and more separate and lost. I tried various ways to anesthetize myself and to escape the desperation I felt. My parents had taught me well one way to do this, but drinking did not feel good. Intellectually, I knew it would degenerate my physical body, and out of pride from the past, I just could not do that to myself.

The philosopher inside me really wanted to understand what was happening in my life. It quickly brought me into an internal conflict that manifested in questions like "Who am I?" "Why am I here?" "What is the purpose of my life?" "How can I feel good about myself if I'm not the best?" "Why is there so much hypocrisy in religion and politics?" "Where are the enlightened people?" "What and where is my path to happiness?"

By asking the questions, I was led to the beginning of learning some answers. Ten days before my eighteenth birthday, I started Transcendental Meditation (TM). At that moment my life changed. My experience was deep — I remembered how to transcend, how to go within myself. I realized that this ability was something I had learned before in other lifetimes, never to forget. One minute I felt the nervousness in my body and my heart pounding in my chest; the next minute I was immersed in a silent body, barely breathing, yet totally awake and aware. It felt so natural and so wonderfully peaceful. I had probably transcended my ego and was experiencing the serenity of spirit. At that moment, there was no intellect asking questions, no ego voice interfering with doubts and discomfort. It was a space of expanding tranquility — a place where everything was OK, totally perfect in the forever moment. I instinctively knew this place of silence. It was not a memory that was being recalled — it was that infinity of Self, our inner connection to the omnipresent divinity, that had always been there. It was the reconnection to Oneness.

As I learned the theory and the practice of the TM program, I realized it fit like a glove with all the ideals and beliefs that had been abstractly floating within me. In my meditation the connections started to be made. I knew from the first day that this was a gift from God and that it would initiate a path of knowledge and catalyze an experience of higher octaves of being.

After two years I decided to go deeper into my understanding of pure consciousness, which by then I had realized was the essence of myself. I studied personally with Maharishi Mahesh Yogi and became a teacher of TM. For ten years, this was the spiritual path I rejoiced in; it has been the most important meditation technique I have practiced.

This meditation connected me with my true Self. It wasn't an intellectual experience, though as a result of inner experiences I learned the dynamics of consciousness, and energy flow within me. Knowing how to transcend, to let go of the outside world, opened infinity into my inner and outer worlds of boundaries. Over the years, my self-discovery unfolded naturally as a result of the practice of meditation and the actual inner cognitions that in time became conscious. I watched my body release its energetic blockages; I felt it normalize through the deep restfulness of silence. I also watched many of the repressed emotions unfold themselves. I had a guru I could trust, who mirrored to me exactly what I needed and gave me the opportunity to teach meditation at the age of twenty. I learned much from all of the people who came to learn the TM technique. Most importantly, I saw how people changed when they started to open to their inner spirit.

As the years passed, my meditation produced peace and calm within me, but I began to realize that it is not enough to find peacefulness — we must also develop the capacity to find joy in it. That ability comes from the process of living and learning the wisdom of peacefulness. It requires us to experience the present moment in its fullness, not just as a fleeting moment of superficial peace; it requires us to know the depth and dignity of spirit and live that moment holistically. I have had a very difficult time learning that lesson because to do so requires experiencing and learning the opposite components, restlessness and disturbance. As these energies surfaced, I became suspect of certain subconscious blockages within me — I intuitively knew there were energies I was not expressing in my life.

This swinging of the pendulum from peace and calm to restlessness and inner disturbance allowed me to move to the next step of my evolution. My developing consciousness was beginning to bring me more in touch with my core emotional themes. The emotional doors locked by my deep denial had begun to open as my meditation took me deeper. But when the energy of my core themes began to flow and manifest, the peace and calm were definitely overshadowed because it was now time to "clean house." A new stage of growth was knocking on the door. For me, it quickly started pounding as my "Saturn Return" approached.

Let me explain. From the time we are born until about 29½ years of age, Saturn is making its long journey around the Sun. When it returns to the position it was in when we were born, this marks one of the most significant astrological time periods in a person's life. Saturn is symbolic of the sometimes harsh school-teacher who is responsible for teaching us our karmic lessons on earth and helping us become the master of living life in harmony and peace. For 28 years we experience life, and if we pay attention and learn, then during "exam" time we will demonstrate our knowledge and graduate to the next level. The Saturn Return is this exam. It is a time to look at our lessons — our karmic issues — and resolve them so that we can move forward in life. But if we've been "asleep," or in denial, or not learning our lessons, the harsh school-teacher calls us to account and makes us work even harder. Most of the time, this makes life difficult and painful.

At around 28 years of age, Saturn approaches the natal position, and we start to feel its influence. The energy increases until it peaks at 29½, and then it gradually fades out by 30½. So for 2½ years we have a chance to learn greatly, to grow quickly, and to move onto a new path of evolution. We have a second Saturn Return at age 59, but the first is usually the most critical one. What occurred for my wife, Paula Kaufman, is an example of just how intense a Saturn Return can be. She experienced the loss of a pregnancy; the loss of the most beloved person in her life, her father; a divorce; a change of career; and living on her own with two young children. But from these difficult experiences came tremendous growth.

As the influence of my own Saturn Return grew, I started to realize that there was more and more inner work to be done. My meditation practice was my constant companion and helper, but it was time to expand, to create new tools, to manifest more resources in my life. I was finally ready to completely confront my deepest denial.

At 28 years old, I found myself in an unfulfilling and inappropriate profession. I had spent three years of working at a design table, struggling through mechanical and solar engineering. Then "out of the blue," I developed a "pain in the neck."

My neck froze up to the point where most of the time I could barely turn my head, and then only with excruciating pain. I could not understand it — my physical health had always been stable and strong. I had never been sick! My life was thrown into confusion and turmoil.

Later I learned what an incredible controller I had always been. I had the ability to hold everything in balance through sheer willpower. But my friend Saturn was ready to shake me up and expose me to a world that I had held under control because of my fear of confronting it: my denial of the "emotional body," the energy field where our emotional energies and the memories that produced them are imprinted and stored. I went to doctors, to chiropractors, to acupuncturists, to massage therapists — you name it — but nothing helped. Some of them said I would have to learn to live with the pain. All of them said they couldn't find a cause — or any reason for the stiff neck.

Of course, this situation created a high degree of anxiety, confusion, and frustration for me. It limited my life to such an extent that it was as if I was being told, "Pay attention! Look deeply into this blockage or it will be with you forever." The amazing thing is that the denial of my emotional issues was so strong that I never suspected what the problem was. As a matter of fact, Paula, who was a good friend at the time and a psychotherapist, told me what the issue was and I immediately dismissed it — I didn't give it a moment of thought. This "pain in the neck" continued into a second year. By the spring of 1983, I was 29½ years old; emotionally I felt like I was going to explode!

One morning while in deep meditation, I had an amazing experience. I heard a voice, loud and clear within me. It told me to get into my car and drive to Santa Fe, New Mexico, a thirteen-hour trip from San Antonio, Texas. Nothing like this had ever happened before, and normally I would have thought that something like this was craziness. But I believed it — I never for a moment doubted the energy behind the voice. It wasn't logical, but I knew it was real. So I called my boss and told him that I had an emergency and needed a few days off from work. I jumped in my car and drove to New Mexico, the "Land of Enchantment." When I arrived, I felt a moment of panic because I wasn't sure what to do next. I realized this was supposed to be some kind of vision quest, but where was I to look?

I sat on a hill watching a sunset of a thousand colors. Just being in such a magical place was worth the drive — Santa Fe felt special, and through its unique vibration and tangible spiritual energy, it was rejuvenating to my soul. With the combination of clear light, refined air, and an elevation of seven thousand feet, I felt closer to heaven, closer to my Self. I knew something wonderful was happening.

I heard about an astrologer who had a good reputation, and I made an appointment. I felt strange going to an astrologer, because at that time in my life I was rather conventional in my attitudes concerning esoterica and spirituality — I would now say I was very opinionated and rigid! My background had been in the sciences and I had been trained to be objective; however, that need for proof and tangible evidence was quickly dissolving. I was desperate — I felt I had to take a chance. The astrology reading was excellent; it made a lot of sense, and it certainly opened me to new possibilities (she said the next two years would transform me!), but it did not even touch upon my neck problem. So the astrologer gave me several names of other "healer types" that I might call.

One of the names was Chris Griscom. I called her and found out that she had just had a cancellation for the next morning. I interpreted this synchronicity as a sign to take this unusual opening in her schedule, even though I had no idea what kind of work she did and wasn't sure I really wanted to know.

At 8:00 the next morning, I drove out into the beautiful desert area south of Santa Fe. I came to the small village of Galisteo and found an old adobe building sitting on the plain, all by itself.

I felt nervous and excited, but when I met Chris I immediately felt accepted. We talked about my life and my neck. She introduced me to an understanding of the emotional body, clarifying the often-used term within the context of her individual style of healing work. She explained that the emotional body holds all the negative emotions such as fear, anger, helplessness, insecurity, etc. Chris also explained how, along with these energies, the emotional body also holds the memories that have produced them — like thick onions, each intense emotional experience contributing another layer to the onion. In order to heal, we have to peel the onion by using our spiritual energy as the healing agent.

I realized then how my emotional body energetically held the imprints of my past experience and structured them within my physical body. My neck became the focus of my attention so that I could get in touch with the blocked emotional energy and the karmic lesson that my "Higher Self" — my "inner knowing," that voice of divinity within — was trying to teach me. But I was completely in the dark as to what that lesson could be. As far as I was concerned, my life had always been perfect. . . .

I climbed nervously onto the massage table. Because of my years of meditation, I knew how to go inside myself. We went through some simple meditation exercises using the healing energy of light, and then I asked inwardly to be shown what was happening inside my emotional body to cause my frozen neck. My Higher Self spontaneously showed me what the karmic theme was and how it had manifested in this lifetime. I was astounded to find that something so obvious was so effectively buried in denial!

I saw that my separation from my mother was caused by a mountain of judgment and blame. I saw how I had closed my heart and withdrawn all communication in our relationship. I felt my anger about her alcoholism and how it had caused self-destruction. Most importantly, I saw how *I* was contributing — how I was feeding the codependency not only with my mother, but also in my other family relationships. My judgment was so intense that all of my attitudes toward her had solidified into the rigidity of iron in my neck muscles. That extreme inner tension of unforgiving anger had created this unyielding, inflexible neck problem.

This particular theme, which I call "separation/judgment," is in my opinion an expression of the deepest karmic theme on the planet—a theme from which only the enlightened are immune and one that will be elaborated upon in detail throughout this book. I see these energies as two aspects of a common energy and inseparable in effect. During that initial session with Chris, I really saw for the first time what separation/judgment was: a powerful emotional energy at the core of the emotional body that actually has a sticky quality, acting like a magnet to attach itself emotionally, especially from an adult child of alcoholic parents to those same parents (in my case, to the parent of the opposite sex).

Through my introduction to this type of emotional-body clearing work, I realized that it is not just by recognizing karmic themes but through actually using the transformative spiritual energy that I could release the attachment of this sticky energy from my consciousness. There was a physical, emotional, mental, and even etheric change that took place, which moved me forward to a *knowing* that could not be denied. I thank Chris for facilitating this peak experience, but as she says, it is the Higher Self—the divine knowing within—that does the work and deserves the credit. From that moment I realized that the plan my Higher Self was following was perfect.

This single experience of self-discovery has become the basis for my spiritual work, which is to not only uncover the hidden energies of the emotional body but also to transmute limitations into boundlessness. This was and is the most rewarding work I have ever experienced.

After that two-hour session, I felt so elated, so expanded, so full of love, especially toward my mother. With the release, there also dawned an understanding of how I had chosen to play the role of victim and how, because of her great love for me, my mother had been willing to play the victimizer in my life. By releasing my judgment of her, I was also giving her an opportunity to free herself from the role. I went home and talked to my parents more openly and truthfully than ever before. It was a tremendous healing. Shortly after that, my mother went into treatment and quit drinking. Though she has relapsed, I am all right. I no longer play the classic codependent, full of judgment and reaction. I have more compassion and understanding. I also realize that she has her own karma to work on and, therefore, she has choice in her life. She must take responsibility for herself, as I am doing for my life.

It was not until about a week after my trip to New Mexico, when I had finally "come back to earth" and settled back into my routine of life, that I realized that there was no more neck pain. As I thought back, I realized that the evening after my session with Chris my neck felt normal again — there was no stiffness, no pain. I was astonished!

It was then I understood that the throat chakra, which controls the neck and shoulders, is where the karmic imprint of separation/judgment is held. As I thought more about the session and what my Higher Self had revealed to me about my life, I saw how separation/judgment had penetrated every aspect of my life, along with its companion self-righteousness, that attitude of "I'm right — you are wrong; this is good and that is bad" — the polarities of the emotional body. Besides realizing that my theme of judgment toward my mother's alcoholism had been the "pain in my neck," I saw more clearly my "rigid" attitudes and my conservative ideas of "shoulds" and "should nots."

Shortly after the miraculous healing of my frozen neck, it became clear that it was time to make a career change. I felt so inspired by the changes in my own life that I wanted to inspire others to help themselves. I plunged into reading everything I could find about metaphysics, and I was soon guided to the area of energetic healing and the concept of subtle bodies of energy.

I decided to quit my job and start training in the traditional systems of healing found in the East; within two years, I completed my training in Chinese medicine (acupuncture and Chinese herbology). The astrologer had been right when she said that the next two years would be transformational! The fuse had been ignited, and I was off and running. . . .

It was evident that the time had come to express my healing potential, which had remained dormant until I could clear away enough of the judgment and related rigidity to allow my healing energy to flow. Once I had done that, the energy did begin to flow! I didn't consciously try to make this happen, but by "letting go," the energy moved spontaneously.

I began to have weekly experiences with kundalini energy, which commonly is felt as a fiery current rising from the base of the spine up through the vertebrae into the head. It can be felt either as a warm flow or as a powerful rocket of energy exploding through the body. It can produce miracles of healing or it can "fry the brain" as it consumes the blood sugar from the brain. The kundalini energy is not something to naively flirt with, but to culture through years of meditation. As a general rule, the more impurity and blockages we have, the less we should open the kundalini. Otherwise, we may short-circuit the nervous system with an energy we are not prepared to handle or risk the flow being obstructed, with detrimental effect. For me, the experiences were very positive, and they have continued regularly until this present time.

Another significant change that occurred during my Saturn Return was in the giving and receiving of love. To put it very simply, I more clearly realized that we are here to love and be loved. I was never very good at that before. I had experienced "love" in the past, but it was always a brief experience and was quickly inhibited. I now had discovered that what I previously thought was love was a sickly, dependent feeling arising from lifetimes of feeling separate and alone. As a result, all my relationships had been dysfunctional and disappointing. I had never understood why my intimate relationships did not last. After I discovered this widespread separation/judgment issue, it was no longer a mystery. What happens when someone judges you? When you judge another? Probably you will "step back," furthering the separation. How can two people be intimate with this separation between them?

After clearing this initial obstacle, it seemed natural for me to draw in a woman whom I could love and be loved by. She was not what I expected. She did not fit the old judgmental "checklist" that I had held in my thick skull, but her spiritual magnetism and unconditional love erased the tapes inside me. I had always been involved with physically beautiful women, and being a "double Libra" didn't help matters: I had the typical attachments and cravings for beauty and perfection. Paula's beauty came from within; she exuded a radiance of love that made people feel at home with themselves. Though I initially resisted her light, my Higher Self helped me heal the illusions of my emotional body. With her love catalyzing the healing within me, I slowly dissolved away my attachment to the superficial. I saw real beauty, which transcends all dimensions. It was my first sight of the archetypal Goddess in human form — the Mother Divine within every woman — with her love that melts all judgment. I felt the truth of the saying "Love is the answer": Paula has been my master teacher.

In the autumn of 1984, after my initial studies in Chinese medicine had been completed, Chris began to train three others and myself in her style of healing work. We had a wonderful but intense training experience! In the middle of the training, Shirley MacLaine wrote *Dancing in the Light*, in which she discussed her past-life memories and experiences with this work. People started calling, and we immediately had clients wanting to experience their Higher Selves and clear their emotional bodies. As a result, the Light Institute was founded in February 1985, and the five of us couldn't begin to handle the demand for sessions. Over the years we added three more facilitators, including Paula.

Paula clearly manifests the Mother Earth energy — she is one of the finest and most powerful healers I've ever witnessed. She brings the infinite power of love with wisdom into this process. Her pragmatic approach plus her 26 years of experience as a counseling and educational psychologist blend beautifully with her psychic gifts, enabling her to penetrate into the heart of the karmic themes. Clients feel safe and secure through a process that can be very emotional and sometimes overwhelming. It is love that brings clients the confidence that they can handle whatever comes to them and the willingness to keep going deeper. Paula exemplifies the true role of a facilitator who does not give the client the "answer," but rather sets up the environment for success and therefore plays a supportive part in the drama of clearing the person's emotional body.

We live in a world of constant change and growth, and at this particular time in history, change can be swift. At the beginning of 1988, after three years of birthing and raising the child we called the Light Institute, it was time for me to break away and manifest a new and expanded dream. I had seen many people learn how to heal themselves through the wisdom of their Higher Self, and it was natural to continue to seek new ways and new technologies that would fit the needs of the individual.

I joined with Paula and two dear friends, Werner Ruoff of Basel, Switzerland, and Peter Evans of Seattle, Washington, to give birth to our own vision, one that would provide multidimensional nourishment to the planet: a nonprofit, charitable, and educational organization whose purpose would be to offer new programs to a world in need. The Deva Foundation became that manifested dream, and it is fulfilling the vision in ways we never anticipated. Through individual sessions, offered to energetically clear the attachments of the emotional body, we assist people in opening the channel to their Higher Self.

For me personally, I have structured an organization and gifted people around me to support my own growth of consciousness. These people are quick to point out any denial or procrastination of purpose I may be experiencing. Therefore, I am helping myself as I help others. At this point in time I am finding that situation to be ideal for fulfilling my life's purpose.

Two

The
Divine
Inner Child

*The law of love could be best
understood and learned through
little children.*

MAHATMA GANDHI

*I*t is amazing where and with
whom we've chosen to incarnate during this lifetime. Sometimes when we look at our family situation, we can wonder
why or even how we chose such a bizarre condition. What we
don't often realize is how fortunate we are to have this opportunity to be in our human bodies and, beyond that, to be in
our human bodies at this time in history — the advent of the
New Age.

Many souls coming in understand their collective purpose,
which is to realize "enlightenment," the expression of full potential, individually and collectively. We have critically important
work to do — there is a reason we are all here right now. The
planetary consciousness has also been evolving, as the souls that
come and go evolve along their chosen paths. Now we have
come to the brink of a glorious time: the majority of souls will

19

shed the maya (illusion) of their perspectives and realize higher levels of harmony and bliss. It can be called the arrival of a state of heaven on earth.

Again, the conventional response may be, "Are you kidding? I didn't choose those parents" or "Why would I want to be born and raised in this place?" or "If this is the dawning of an age of enlightenment, what would an age of ignorance be like?" There is superficial validity to these questions, but we cannot look at the surface value of life any longer. The answer lies deeper, below the surface, beyond the mind: inside the individual's heart. It lies in the dream — the collective dream — that we are manifesting. Evolution is progressive, and we are learning our lessons. We are gaining wisdom, no matter how scattered and fragmented the process seems to be. Now is the time to pull it into coherence — for the pieces of the cosmic puzzle to fall into a clear picture.

This process doesn't start outside — it begins inside and expands outward. Expansion implies a movement from less to more, from seed to flower. If we look only at the surface of life, we miss almost everything. So we must again look at the deepest values of life, and then we must closely examine our birth in this lifetime — or in any lifetime — because birth is symbolic of a new beginning but also of the separation from the Mother. So with our birth, we start to learn and grow once again from our deepest lesson: separation.

What is the deepest, most fundamental aspect of ourselves? What did God create first? That reflection of God within the boundaries of individual consciousness but connected to the infinite is what we call the soul. The soul is immortal, unchanging, infinite in its scope, yet it can breathe life into the finite. It is the reflection of God within us. The soul's consciousness is the consciousness of God, and therefore it is infinite and eternal. When we live in conscious contact with the soul, we realize cosmic consciousness, an all-inclusive state of consciousness where the awareness of our soul, or our Inner Self, is never lost

— it becomes the witness to waking, dreaming, and sleep states of consciousness.

The voice of the soul, the wisdom of our God-nature, expresses itself through what we can call the Higher Self, our divine knowing, the hologram of who we are. The Higher Self bridges the infinite with the finite. It communicates the pure knowledge of the soul to all of the "subtle bodies," those coexisting energetic aspects of our multidimensional nature. The Higher Self is our guide and master teacher in each lifetime, whether we know it consciously or not. It knows every moment and every choice in every lifetime. The more conscious we become, the clearer the Higher Self manifests its guidance and knowing in our life.

All of our choices and experiences are recorded in the great "cosmic computer," commonly known as the Akashic Records. This "other-dimensional computer" records the soul's long journey through its incarnations but *not* the emotional content of the life experiences. This means that the actions taken in our life are listed there, but the subtle feelings and emotions underlying these actions are not. The Higher Self, however, knows it all — everything about us, inside and out. Like the computer expert, the Higher Self can access information from the Akashic Records as well as from the imprints of the emotional body. So it can be our fastest path to the realization of Self, the 24-hour-a-day consciousness of our essential nature.

There are different masks the Higher Self can wear as it appears to us inwardly. Usually these masks are symbolic. But the easiest aspect for us to work with is the form that appears at the beginning of our incarnation. The energy of the Higher Self that comes into the body first is what I call the "Divine Child," to be distinguished from the concepts of the "Inner Child" or the "Child Within" commonly used in psychotherapy. The physical form of the child is different from the wise, knowing form of our symbolic Inner Child. Therefore, *the Divine Child is a dimension or an aspect of our Higher Self*, and like other aspects of the Higher Self, the symbol enriches us with its unique hologram of possibilities and unique perspectives.

If we take the point of view expressed in reincarnation theories, the soul manifests a physical body, lives the life, drops the body, moves into a transition period in a spirit body, and then comes back into another body; this process is repeated over and over again. During the transition period, we have time to evaluate what has happened in the previous lifetime and review our karmic path. It's a time to look at what we've accomplished and what remains to be learned. At that moment, the Higher Self is making the choices for creating our next incarnation. We choose our parents, where we will be born, the period in history, what karmic issues we will work on through our experiences of that lifetime, and what the priorities will be; we then structure all of this into a loose outline of possibilities. This structure is not fixed, but flexible and adaptable to the changes we experience in life. So at any point in time we can shift the path. Usually we don't shift it dramatically, but through the success of working through our karmic attachments we may find a more efficient pathway or we may get stuck on some tangent that requires more time to process a particular issue. We are always moving forward in the evolutionary process, with the experiences of each present moment influencing what we call "future" in this loose outline of possibilities.

When we are ready, we transit the dimensions into the physical body of a baby. The spiritual energy of the Higher Self that leads us at this time is the Divine Child. This is the spirit that infuses the body with the knowing of our divinity.

This concept is quite different from the common idea of the Inner Child used in psychotherapy. Many therapists work with the Inner Child but see its expression as an aspect of the emotional body. This means that they are accessing memories and feelings of childhood for the purpose of clearing the earlier building blocks of current emotional problems. While it is true that many times the Inner Child appears distressed, full of pain and separation, I would interpret this for what it really is: the overshadowing influence of the karmic themes of the emotional body. The Inner Child mirrors those issues we need to resolve within ourselves and encourages us to take action so that we can relate to that unique part of ourselves.

If a therapist sees the Inner Child only as an effective technique that symbolically reveals emotional themes, there may be some benefit, but those benefits may be only a small portion of what potentially might be achieved. When the therapist views the Inner Child as a creation of the emotional body that mirrors the negative memories and feelings of childhood, this point of view limits the client. It is a limitation because the therapist continues to work on the level of the emotional body instead of accessing the higher vibration of the Divine Child Within to release the *source* of our emotional attachments.

If the therapist knows that the Divine Child is all-knowing, a reflection of God in the body of a baby, then no matter what the overshadowing situation may be, he or she will help the client to access the deeper answer, and the solution can be manifested. The point of view of the therapist is crucial.

The techniques and approach are, of course, important, but the spiritual perspective has a powerful effect on the client and, therefore, on the expression of the Inner Child. Otherwise, the illusion of the emotional body is perpetuated, and that maya blocks us from our divinity. The alternate perspective says, "I am not my karma. I am not my fear, loneliness, anger, etc. I am the Sun, not the clouds that may temporarily overshadow it."

When I first heard about the Inner Child, I considered it a clever technique to access the emotional imprints of childhood. I proceeded to be instructed in some different ways to work with the Inner Child, but at that time they were just "practice" sessions. I did not see anything spiritual about the process — to me, it was just another emotional technique.

Several months later, in sessions with my first "real" clients, I noticed that something else was happening. Instead of the client simply accessing wounded-child feelings, I felt the entrance into our joint consciousness of a quality of light and healing that was as tangible as if someone had turned on a thousand floodlights. The Divine Child came forth as a vibrant awareness of wisdom that immediately guided the client through the healing of childhood wounds. This phenomenon is not some contrived technique to work on emotions but is an aspect of our inner divinity that is utterly real. As this experience was repeated continually over a few months, I decided it was time to get on the massage table and experience my own Divine Child.

At first I was disappointed, because what I experienced was not what I expected but rather a plunging into childhood memories. I seemed to be like so many others. I needed to clear old feelings of sadness and loneliness. Toward the end of my session, however, I felt a distinct shift in the energy flow of my body, like a feeling of being nurtured. That feeling remained without being overshadowed by any of the other feelings.

Several weeks later I did another session with the Inner Child. This time I felt like a different person. Though my intention was to continue to clear and balance my emotions, especially regarding my childhood, this time the Child appeared in a different form. He was radiant! It was obvious that I was experiencing a completely different energy, an energy of pure spirit. There was not a trace of judgment. On the contrary, I felt omnipresent unity. I knew I *was* that child. This Divine Child held in his presence a peace and a knowing that brought buckets of tears out of me. These tears, however, were of a happiness and joy that I had never felt before. At that moment, my inner knowing communicated to me in a few seconds the understanding of how to help people access and understand their own Divine Child. I had made the quantum leap from the sometimes-empty memorization of a psychological technique to the artistic richness of being a facilitator of this form of the Higher Self. Through my learning from clients plus my own personal experience, I have since developed several approaches to working with the Divine Child.

A basic example that I've witnessed several times in the last few years follows.

One of my new clients had spent three years working weekly with a psychoanalyst. At least forty of those sessions had been spent working with his wounded Inner Child. In each session the wounded child dredged up more and more pain — every variation of the helpless victim, a child held powerless by the frightening world around him. Over the years my client became increasingly frustrated with these sessions, and the obvious questions arose: "Will I ever heal this child? Is the pain unlimited?"

Of course, when I suggested we work with the Divine Child, he was ready to run for the door! But my different point of view and his willingness to seek a spiritual answer were enough to clear the pain of the emotional body. He became free of his indulgence of the emotional body, an addiction to creating and perpetuating the wounded child ad infinitum. He gave himself permission to experience a beautiful and wonderful dimension of his Higher Self that had been blocked to his awareness before, one that provided an energy that could heal his wounds.

It is common these days to be instructed to plunge into the pain — to feel it and overcome it. Many times we feel better after hours of crying, and intellectually we want to believe that it was worth the effort. But there is a difference between indulging in our pain and releasing the energy of attachment to the pain. By swimming in it, we may just perpetuate it with no release of the attachment in the emotional body. By radiating the light and love of the Higher Self, we dissolve energetically the karmic connection, and the pain we experience is the pain moving outward, being released. This is a true release, an energetic change that transforms us, that clears another cloud from the sun.

This man was amazed to find that in one session he was able to resolve more than he had in forty sessions with his psychoanalyst. He was convinced that the spiritual approach opened him to an authentic healing and, at the same time, an understanding — we could call it an "inner knowing" — that provided a lesson that will never be forgotten and a wisdom that continually grows pragmatically in life.

The Inner Child also relates to our attitudes and feelings about children. Since childhood is a vulnerable time of life, our childhood experience can be full of traumatic memories and deeply imprinted emotional issues. The presence of these heavy energies can bias our attitudes and feelings toward our own children or toward children in general. A woman who has had a painful childhood may avoid having her own children for fear that the situation will repeat itself or elicit old buried feelings that cause discomfort. The possibilities are numerous, and the healing can be difficult. Again, the Divine Child knows the necessary remedy and will provide us the opportunity for its use.

In our work I find that this situation commonly arises, and I always marvel at the genius of the Divine Child in its effectiveness of resolution. Three years ago I was working with a woman who was desperately trying to get pregnant, but to no avail. She and her husband had been to the best physicians, had participated in endless laboratory tests to find the problem to her infertility or conception difficulty. For years nothing had proved helpful. She suspected there must be an emotional issue at the basis of her problem, but after six months of therapy all she had gained was a better understanding of a miserable childhood. By the time she was referred to me she was panicked, because she was in her late thirties and felt she was getting too old to conceive.

In her first session, her Divine Child appeared as a radiant, blue Krishna child, floating above her with a big smile on his face. The Child took her back to a memory in a past life where she was pregnant and died with her child while giving birth, alone in the corner of an old barn stall. Before she died, immersed in the pain and intense sadness of defeat, she had sworn that she would never again attempt childbirth. It was not the physical pain that prompted this but the guilt she felt about having failed and having killed the baby. That oath she promised imprinted the emotional body with the guilt, the pain — the hologram of her suffering about childbirth — and started a series of lifetimes where a variation on this theme perpetuated itself into the present time.

The beautiful part of the session was the love that her Divine Child demonstrated while he unfolded the memories for her. She felt surrounded by a compassion and healing light that removed her pain, and the tears that flowed were tears of relief and transformation. Her Divine Child guided her through the crucial moments, giving advice and support that encouraged her to move forward and gave her the strength to let go.

As the facilitator, I felt a beautiful blue-violet presence, comforting yet stimulating to every atom in the room. Her body went through muscle spasms and hot and cold spells as the energies of the past moved out of her. It was a powerful experience to witness.

After a period of rest to stabilize her bodily and emotional reactions, we discussed her experience, and it was obvious that she was now a different woman. She knew it, too. The conclusion of the story is that she called me three weeks later to tell me she was pregnant.

To the skeptical reader, these examples may sound like fanciful stories of a magic touch or a secret formula. But these successes are simply the result of individuals opening their own spiritual potential and channeling that infinite power into their blockages of life. If this is magic, then it is the divine magic that we all own and now can learn to trust. In the simple and natural is the infinite power of God.

It is important to understand that if the Divine Child is an aspect of the Higher Self, then it has the knowing of the Higher Self. Therefore, the Child knows your karmic choices for this lifetime and also knows about the early building blocks of current emotional problems. You can trust the Child as you would trust your Higher Self. You can ask questions and get answers. The Child is not a spirit guide or some entity coming through — it is *you*, straightforward, so humanly divine, so simple, yet so wise. . . .

In my practice, I have found that one of the easiest ways to introduce clients to their Higher Self is to start by contacting their Divine Child. What follows is a common experience I relate to clients to exemplify this concept.

I wake up one morning depressed, cloudy, and confused. My first thoughts are, Why do I feel this way? and What can I do to feel better? It would seem intelligent to ask inside for the answer or at least a clue as to what is happening. So, I ask the Higher Self. If I'm clear, I may channel through a lengthy answer on the nature of my karmic themes and how these themes impinge upon my consciousness now, because of various choices already made and the optimum timing to experience them. . . .

Well, if you've ever been in a depression, you know that you may not particularly care about all of this "stuff," whether it is correct or not. So another approach to this situation is to ask the Divine Child to help you. Very quickly it tells you that the reason you are depressed is that you haven't had any fun today — the perfect words because they are so simple and to the point, while at the same time the solution to the problem. The Inner Child has a way of bypassing the "mind body" — that linear, primarily "left-brain" intellectual aspect of mind — and with simplicity releases the crippling energy surrounding us. In the situation described above, asking the Child can provide the answers you are seeking in the simplest and most direct way.

The Child brings in a point of view that is very helpful for the adult — there are qualities of the Child that we tend to lose or push aside as we "grow up." The Child reminds us how to live in the moment. Children have no concept of past or future — they are new to this world and therefore "past" has not accumulated yet. They have no memories to speak of or to feel bad about (except possibly their birth) and no worries about what might happen tomorrow. So children can be in the here and now. Remember that the Inner Child has just come from a dimension of timelessness and therefore brings that energy into this world.

It is wonderful to see people after they have worked with their

Divine Child in our Deva sessions, and how they manifest that Divine Child energy into their life. They start to enjoy living in the moment as the Child becomes more visible. This quality of being here and now may be one of the most important qualities that we can master. It frees us from the grip of time by opening the door to the inner world, where time does not exist. The Divine Child leads us to the world of spirit and oneness.

The Child remembers "the other side," where experience is holographic, not linear. This multidimensionality is the norm for the Divine Child. Intuition, or "right-brain function," is naturally open because the aspect of linear time is not impacting our current reality. Therefore, the Divine Child or Higher Self quality is infused with this unbounded awareness, which can act as a complement for the mind body's need to live in a world of relative time and space. The spiritual transcendent becomes integrated into time and space, and we can flow with it but not be attached to it. The Divine Child has that invaluable knowing. As an adult, we tend to be drawn to the rational, intellectual point of view of the mind body, often to an excess. An occasional touch of the Divine Child's magic can open the feminine, abstract, non-linear, artistic, intuitional right-brain function of that very same mind body. In a world of such masculine focus, this can be a saving grace!

Another quality of the Divine Child is the ability to experience simple joys. A small child does not need sophistication, complexity, or a lot of stimulus. He or she can be fascinated with simple pleasures and a simple life, while at the same time there is an innate need to expand, to grow, to break boundaries. The child has come in to live life, to experience all things. It is programmed with the energy of the Higher Self and wants to expand into the infinite — it is curious to know all things. We have this impulse at the beginning of each lifetime. How long it stays vital within us is dependent on our situation. Unfortunately, the older we get the more it usually fades. Our Inner Child can help remedy that problem by rejuvenating us with the evolutionary force.

The small child has innocence, which is a wonderful quality, especially for adults. It is that attitude toward life that is without judgment or guilt, yet is not naive. Innocence implies a spiritual knowing that is in harmony with nature and trusts the universe. The innocence of a child can express itself in its acceptance of the order of all things as being naturally perfect.

Another characteristic, and a most important one, is that children know how to play and how to have fun, naturally and spontaneously. This genius manifests in their ability to use the simple elements of life in a refreshing and creative manner to entertain and live the joy in the moment. It's unfortunate that most adults have forgotten how to have simple fun without a shot of potent stimulation. The natural creativity of the Divine Child allows us to be expansive and progressive in our play, without the attachment or addiction that causes limitation or the feeling that "this is the only way to feel good." The qualities of the Child encourage expansion, not stagnation; creativity, not routine; naturalness, not conventionality. Most people are in need of nourishment, and the play of the Divine Child manifesting through the adult is a great place to start.

Lastly, the Divine Child can provide much humor and laughter to us all. It has no need for seriousness and heaviness. How can you play and have fun with seriousness weighing you down? Feel the smile of the Divine Child uplift you and your world.

The emergence of the Divine Child will occur naturally as we clear the blockages to our self-knowledge. When the judgments and separation fall away, the Divine Child is present in all its glory. We will feel the integration of spirit into the material world. We will feel the freedom of the true Self, with no need for attachment and no need for denial of our humanness. The Divine Child is spirit integrated into the human form. It holds the infinite potential of both forms, available here and now.

By choosing to work with the Divine Child, we select a communication channel that is simple and has a heart. The Higher

Self doesn't have to appear as God standing on a cloud surrounded by angels, giving some earth-shattering message. In fact, I don't know many people who experience the Higher Self that way. The communication from our inner knowing may be subtle — a whisper, an intuitive feeling, a symbol, a word, a synchronistic event; it may come instantly or later from a dream, or as a surprise while we are washing the dishes. One thing that will help is to be *awake* and *open* . . . to be like the Child.

Many therapists have worked with the Inner Child through different approaches and with different interpretations of experience. In our work, the Inner Child is an aspect or dimension of the Higher Self and therefore is *real*. Our interpretation is that we are multidimensional beings. That means we have many aspects, many levels of knowledge, and many perspectives of expression that are integrated into a wholeness. Everyone would agree that we have a physical body because it is tangible. However, our other aspects, which can be called our subtle bodies, are just as real. During an out-of-body experience, we can know the reality of a spirit body, for example, which then shifts our perspective and, therefore, our sense of reality. To truly know the Self is to perceive and utilize all of our dimensions, to bring expanded consciousness to the hologram that we are. The experience and understanding of our subtle bodies helps accomplish the purpose of self-discovery.

Anyone who works in this area of subtle-body balancing starts to realize that the inner world is more "real" than the outer world, because the energy is more powerful, more infinite in nature. On the level of the subatomic, infinity is the rule, death the exception — there are protons and neutrons that are billions of years old. Etheric and other subtle energies are immortal.

This is another example of how the deeper levels of life are more lasting, less changeable than the superficial levels of life. There is more orderliness, greater coherence of form and function. When our attention is fixed only on the superficial level, we become identified with that dimension and tend to make judgments based on a limited perspective. It is such an expansion to look deeper, to finally appreciate the infinite values, to release ourselves from singular viewpoints and enjoy the whole. It may be temporarily enjoyable to play the piano with one finger, and we may develop to our full capacity in performing this task, but what about playing the piano with ten fingers? Then we are ready to join the symphony orchestra. It's time to open to our full potential!

Three

Multidimensionality & Our Subtle Bodies

Why do I seem to be in so many places at the same time?
CLIENT

How can I feel like I'm in two places at once and at the same time feel like I'm no place at all?
CLIENT

*P*repare *yourself for a journey into the mind body. . . . Understand that the following may cause symptoms of drowsiness, disoriented thinking, and such questions as "Why do I need to know this?" or "What does this have to do with the Divine Child?" If you experience these symptoms, don't be concerned. Just get up and run around the room and then keep reading. . . .*

After many years of studying Chinese medicine and Ayurvedic medicine, the ideas of energetic bodies became more clear to me. Bodies of energy more subtle than our material physical body can begin to be investigated and subjectively experienced through practices of acupuncture, energetic herbal remedies, and aspects of yoga. When we combine the information gained with the data bank of psychic/spiritual experiences, we open a door to a new world of possibilities for understanding ourselves.

A "subtle body," by definition, is not something physically material that we can see and touch but rather a field of energy that coexists with our physical body, yet in another dimension of reality. We use the word "subtle" because these other energetic bodies exist in a dimension beyond normal perception and seem to be transcendental to the physical world. The different dimension is due to a different vibratory rate of energy. Subtle bodies all coexist simultaneously with the physical body — they are not separate, but fully integrated into the totality of who we are.

Subtle bodies have been given various names, but those we will use here are "emotional body," "astral body," "etheric body," "mind body," and "spiritual body." (I've heard a gamut from "galactic body" to "atomic body"!) From the experience of each subtle body comes a unique point of view of reality, a particular quality of energy, and unique qualities of expression of this subtle energy. The subtle bodies are different aspects of our holographic multidimensional nature. As our consciousness expands, our ability to perceive and know the different aspects of the Self becomes clearer. The following analogy can be useful in helping to understand the concept of subtle bodies.

Imagine that we have a "supertuner," similar to a radio tuner, but one that can tune in to the full range of electromagnetic energy frequencies. Not only can we tune in to the radio band, but we can also tune into higher frequencies, such as X-rays, gamma rays, and so on. The tuner has the ability to adjust to any frequency of energy and experience its unique "point of view" or "body" of information. Each of these frequencies may serve a different purpose from other "stations" we may tune into. Radio stations, for example, provide us auditory experience; television stations provide us auditory and visual experience; X-ray stations can be used to study the structure of matter, or to take photographs of the internal condition of our physical bodies. Yet all these "stations" coexist simultaneously within the range of lower-to-higher energy vibration. Though the qualities of the X-ray spectrum are quite different from those of the radio-wave or television-wave spectrums, the only fundamental difference is that of their vibratory rates. Inherent within each vibration, however, is a unique world of information and possibilities of expression.

Within the nonphysical dimension of subtle bodies, there also exists a range of energy frequencies, each with its own purpose, from that of the astral body on the lower end of the spectrum to the spiritual body on higher. The vibrations of the emotional body, for example, are quite different from those of the mind body or the etheric body. And each subtle body has its own unique "subset," if you will, of diverse energy frequencies.

Our "tuner" in this case is our consciousness. However, the key to accessing the subtle frequencies of the energetic world lies in the quality of the tuner — in other words, the more conscious we are, the better "reception" we will get, the less static we will receive.

Let us liken the emotional body to the radio-wave band of our electromagnetic spectrum of energy. Just as on a radio we can tune in to different stations, either AM or FM, each at a different frequency and with a different music format, such as classical, jazz, country, or rock 'n' roll, so in the emotional body we can "tune in" with our consciousness to different emotions, each with its unique quality of energy and its characteristics of emotional expression.

People who have the ability to read "auras" (the energy field that emanates from the etheric body and surrounds the physical body) actually see these vibrations in terms of color. They may commonly see envy, for example, as a dirty-green vibration and judgment as a dirty-indigo vibration. While there is a definite difference between the energies of green and indigo, if we tune into the yellow frequencies, we may see a close relationship between certain emotions, for example, fear and cowardice. These emotions have a similar vibration, and, consequently, they are both dirty yellow in color, though of a slightly different shade. As we experience different emotions, our consciousness is tuning in, so to speak, to different octaves of the emotional body.

The mind body, too, has its own band of energy frequencies. The quality of the vibrations of the linear, dualistic logic of the intellect, for example, is quite different from that of what is called the "higher mind," the highest vibration of the mind body, which knows truth and brings clarity to intuition and choice. This range of frequencies from the slower vibrations to the higher vibrations is true for the other subtle bodies as well.

For example, scientists have shown that certain meditation and yogic practices can produce greater coherence and orderliness in the functioning of the brain, and therefore they bring greater clarity and efficiency to the thinking process. On the contrary, it is obvious that if our brain activity is chaotic, our thinking and action will also be chaotic. If our consciousness (the supertuner) is full of static or interference, then our ability to perceive information and experience will be limited. So the first step of improvement must be to fine-tune the consciousness so that we can receive clear signals. This fine-tuning process will result in greater coherence and orderliness, not only in the brain, but also in all of the subtle bodies. As the orderliness of function improves, the power of our consciousness increases, just as if we are boosting the power of our supertuner so it can capture higher and higher frequencies of energy. Because the highest frequencies of energy bring us to the spiritual body octaves, we find that our tuner is now receiving spiritual energies in greater quantity and quality of experience. Not only will the mind body experience greater understanding and knowledge, but the other subtle bodies will express their spiritual aspects also.

Our analogy with the supertuner and its "stations" goes only so far, however. Whereas different radio stations along the radio band may not directly interrelate with each other — nor with the television or X-ray stations the tuner can pull in — the various subtle bodies do affect each other. In fact, their "tuner" — what we have called consciousness — is not only able to tune in to the various vibrational qualities, it also acts as the "cosmic glue" that holds all of them together. Consciousness is the omnipresent foundation wherein the range of energies exist and interrelate together.

This connection is experienced to a greater or lesser degree depending on the person and his or her degree of consciousness, but it is becoming increasingly evident that, for example, both the emotional body and the mind body affect the physical body — our "attitudes" and emotional responses can lead to changes in our physical well-being, for better or worse.

The mind body can affect our emotional body as well. If we *think* that snakes are harmful, for example, we will experience *fear* when we encounter one. Alternatively, if we *think* of snakes as a symbol of transformation or the continuity of life, we may take their appearance as a good omen and be *delighted* by seeing one.

In conventional medicine and therapy, we commonly see practitioners treating the physical body or mind body, but seldom do we see a holistic approach to treatment that works multi-dimensionally. It is possible to treat the physical and have it affect our other aspects, but usually the effect is minor and inappropriate. My favorite analogy uses the example of a sick plant, whose leaves are turning yellow and whose branches are drooping from weakness. The common approach would be to treat the symptoms, which in this case might mean painting the leaves green and propping up the branches with poles and string. This may improve the superficial appearance of the plant, but it is doubtful that it will improve its health — it may even hasten its demise. The intelligent gardener, on the other hand, knows that you must treat the root of the problem to bring about true healing. Therefore, the gardener waters the root, and immediately all aspects of the plant are healed. For human beings, the "root" or source of our subtle bodies is consciousness. As we nourish and expand our consciousness, the spiritual energy flows into our multidimensional nature, and all aspects of our being are brought into balance and harmony.

Recently, some physicists and physicians have been contributing a new point of view that helps to bridge the gap between subjective experiences and scientific theories of natural law. The physician Dr. Richard Gerber, in his book *Vibrational Medicine*, does an excellent job of interfacing theories of subtle energetic bodies with new ideas in physics. Dr. Gerber discusses the theory of Dr. William Tiller, a physicist who has offered new ideas about the physical laws of the universe. Dr. Tiller's ideas may help to explain the existence of subtle bodies. He refers to two important divisions of existence, the domain of positive space/time and the domain of negative space/time. (Positive and negative do not imply a moralistic judgment of "good" and "bad" but rather refer to a polarity of charge.)

In his theory, Dr. Tiller refers to positive space/time as the material dimension consisting of matter that vibrates at less than the speed of light. This is our common physical space/time universe. The world as we know it is made of matter and energy, linked by the famous Einsteinian equation, $E=mc^2$, in which E represents energy, m represents mass, and c represents the velocity of light. Energy and matter are related by the vibratory rate of light. Therefore, we can say that matter is light that has been "frozen," or that has *slowed down* in vibration until it has "precipitated" into matter. This is not so different from steam condensing first into water as it cools and then into ice (which technically is a slowing down of the molecular vibration of H_2O). Just as energy has different frequencies of vibration, matter also has different frequencies of vibration. The faster the vibration of matter, the closer to light energy we get. Einstein's formula placed an upper limit to the velocity of matter; he thought that nothing could exceed the velocity of light.

Dr. Tiller, however, has introduced a theory of negative space/time in which there exist energies that vibrate faster than light. This theory describes our subtle bodies as existing in negative space/time, which has the following characteristics:

1. It is magnetic in nature;

2. It is a field of negative entropy (a field of coherence and orderliness);

3. It consists of energy that vibrates faster than light;

4. It coexists with positive space/time.

The physical body exists in positive space/time. It obeys the laws of physics and is well understood by modern medicine as far as anatomy and physiology are concerned. But the physical body is only a part of, and is not separate from, our multidimensional nature. We have other "bodies" or energetic forms integrated and coexisting within and around the physical body.

Such forms of healing as acupuncture, meditation and mental techniques, the use of energetic herbs, etc., move beyond the treatment of the physical body and affect the energetic basis of our positive space/time body. The electromagnetic field that we call the "etheric body" is the bridge between positive space/time and negative space/time; it connects the physical body with our other subtle bodies. Because the etheric body is this bridge, it acts as a conduit to take energy from the physical body to the subtle bodies and vice versa, allowing a constant flow of energy back and forth.

The healing system of acupuncture is one example of how we can treat the subtle energy of the etheric body and cause healing to a physical-body problem. Simply put, the metallic acupuncture needles are placed in the appropriate anatomical locations of the physical body that correspond to the etheric body's subtle-energy pathways. The stimulation of energy flow moves through the etheric body and affects a change in the subtle bodies. Then the energy from our subtle bodies immediately flows back through the conduit of the etheric body, producing a corresponding balancing or healing effect on the physical-body condition. This is an example of energetic healing, or what Dr. Gerber calls "vibrational medicine." The etheric body and its energetic pathways always play a key role in the healing of our multidimensional Self.

The etheric body is made up of seven main energy centers called "chakras." These are connected by the median acupuncture meridians, or energy conduits, of the physical body: the conception vessel, which lies on the frontal side, and the governor vessel, which moves through the spinal cord on the back side. Each chakra actually rotates or "spins" at a different rate; therefore, they are seen as emitting different colors. The chakras are connected to each other by subtle-energetic channels, which can be seen as deep acupuncture meridians, but in India are called *nadis*. These nadi channels parallel the body's nerve pathways abundantly: There are 72,000 of these etheric channels!

Since the etheric body is the electromagnetic structure that links the physical body to the other subtle bodies via the "chakra-nadi-acupuncture-meridian" system, it also channels the complete spectrum of higher and lower frequencies within its structure. The lower-vibratory astral body coexists with the higher-vibratory spiritual body within the subtle energetic system.

The acupuncture meridians, which follow well-mapped pathways in the human body, carry a subtle energy that traditionally the Chinese call *ch'i* (pronounced chee) and in India is called *prana*. It is this energy that flows between the subtle bodies and the physical body.

This life-force subtle energy is not uniform, but is always changing depending on the environment in which it is flowing and the qualities of that environment it is reflecting. Ch'i also expresses itself with slightly different mixtures of yin and yang, those essential feminine and masculine energies, respectively, that are the foundation of traditional Chinese philosophy. For example, the ch'i of the yin organ liver is qualitatively different from the ch'i of the yang organ stomach; the ch'i of the aura (primarily yang) is different from the ch'i of our ancestral energy (primarily yin). Ch'i can be diagnosed in this positive space/time world, but it is not limited to this world. It can bridge the different dimensions and octaves of our being. It links the vast potential of our negative-space/time subtle bodies with the human world of form. Unfortunately, our present medical and techno-logical expertise is still not refined enough to be able to measure and systematically describe this world of subtle energy and, therefore, our various subtle bodies, but hopefully that day is not too far off.

The etheric body serves as a multidimensional, holographic energy template that acts as a guide to the creation and forma-tion of the physical body. We can think of it as a manifestation of the Higher Self's methodology for creating the body according to the needs of a person's karmic lessons and, therefore, the needs of the emotional body to structure aspects of itself into matter.

In Chinese medicine there are various diagnostic techniques to determine the condition of the ch'i and, therefore, of the etheric body. The more commonly used diagnostic techniques include a thorough interview with the client, followed by an evaluation of his or her responses based on traditional Chinese medical philosophy, which over thousands of years has produced a beau-tiful system that blends pragmatic physical and emotional infor-mation with a philosophical system of life and living. One tech-nique is the age-old system of pulse diagnosis, which analyzes the quality, quantity, and flow of etheric energy within the meridian system. This system is very similar to the Ayurvedic pulse-diagnosis techniques used in India, also for thousands of years. Various forms of visual and ta tile study of the physical body are used as well.

All of these diagnostic techniques are evaluated and cross-checked, and as the pieces of the puzzle fall together, a picture appears that reveals the person's energetic situation. Skilled practitioners can pinpoint a weakness or imbalance in the etheric body days, weeks, or even months before it is seen physically as a problem. Then they can utilize their preferred system of vibrational medicine to remedy the source right away, rather than having to wait until the future to deal with its expressed symptoms. There are many reliable systems of healing, but my experience has shown that the system from China is one of the best, and its success lies in its understanding and treatment of the energetic bodies.

Our work at the Deva Foundation uses a process similar to that of Chinese medicine, but instead of the facilitator diagnosing and treating the client, *it is the client's own Higher Self that exposes the problem, and it is the Higher Self that implements the remedy.* It is beautiful to watch the intuitional wisdom of the Higher Self provide the answers for the complex of problems that arise in the sessions. Sometimes it is as if our Higher Self were a master physician/healer multidimensionally taking care of us.

To better understand the Higher Self, it is important to understand "where it lives." Its environment is the infinite sea of pure being, that impersonal or abstract aspect of the omnipresent God-energy. The soul is our personal channel, which experiences the waves of God-love in that universal sea of being, as a person who has been still in a hot bath suddenly moves and feels the waves of warmth. The soul can experience unboundedness within the boundaries of its experience; it can know anything within the wisdom of the infinite. It is the *personal* channel from the omnipotence of God into the boundary of each soul's realm of experience, which may run the gamut of the specific to the infinite. It is common to use the term Higher Self as the voice or expression of the soul.

The Higher Self is the epitome of the spiritual body, which according to Dr. Tiller exists in negative space/time and is of the highest vibration. I would add that the spiritual body is not a distinct subtle body like the mind body or emotional body, but rather it includes that portion of the highest vibration of all the subtle bodies. For example, the "higher mind" is the highest vibration of the mind body; the "higher emotional body" is the highest vibration of the emotional body; and the etheric and physical bodies also have a high vibratory connection to the spiritual body.

But the whole is greater than the sum of the parts. The spiritual body is also beyond and between the physical and subtle bodies. The spiritual body is a reflection of God, and God is omnipresent and transcendental. Pure consciousness is the energy of the spiritual body, and therefore all spiritual bodies are unified into the Oneness — one God, one spirit, one consciousness. Because the Higher Self is initially viewed as personal, there is a tendency to call it our own: It is something that is "me" but not "you." As consciousness evolves and expands, we eventually realize, in our enlightenment, that all Higher Selves are one.

One aspect of the spiritual body is the higher mind, that faculty of intellectual wisdom married to intuitional wisdom. We can view it as the balancing and synchronous activity of the right and left brains interfacing with the negative-space/time energies, thus producing a wholeness of mind. The higher mind is the connection to truth and understanding, that knowledge that is specific to the individual's needs at any particular moment.

Another aspect of the spiritual body is the higher emotional body, which is experienced whenever the higher emotional virtues — joy, rapture, ecstasy, bliss, and, of course, the unifying experience of love — are expressed. These higher emotions are the experiential facets of Self, the vibrations of the divine. These feelings are available to everyone and can be felt as we ascend beyond the clouds of the "lower emotional body," which is dominated by such emotions as fear, anger, and jealousy. Through the experience of these higher vibrational energies, we begin to stabilize the emotional body. On these high levels of vibration and through the quickening of the vibration of the lower emotional body, the dense, slow vibrations of our karmic attachments release. Anger, fear, sadness, or any other emotional theme cannot hold on to an emotional body that is vibrating on the level of love and bliss.

Another way of viewing this vibrational shift in the emotional-body spectrum is by looking at the underlying "background energy." Do we have a lot of emotional background "noise," or "static," which is then our platform for. experience? Does the noise trigger a response in our environment that attracts more noise to us, like a magnetic attraction? Or do we have an emotional background energy of peace, joy, and happiness, which attracts more of what we enjoy? The latter case is what we are aiming for, because it is the nature of human beings to seek more and more of the God vibration, though our addictions to the lower vibrations may temporarily hold our attention.

We should not despair over our "lower emotions." As I will discuss later, it is possible to transform the negative aspects into positive, growth-producing experiences that move us quickly into higher energies. For example, by releasing the karmic theme of the abuse of power, we can arrive at a situation where we still have power, but without the "victimizer" running the show. By learning our karmic lessons, we grow. The emotional body plays a leading role in the drama of becoming fully human, that special experience of becoming the master of the heart, the teacher of love and life.

The lowest frequency of the emotional-body spectrum lies in the astral dimension; therefore, the emotional body can be said to be split in two. It is part of the "astral body," but the higher-frequency portion, the higher emotional body, is vibrating within the spiritual body. The astral body is the slowest vibration in negative space/time. It can be experienced in two ways, most commonly as the lower emotional body, which is evidenced by the karmic mask we wear in each lifetime and its expressed emotional themes. The astral body can also be perceived during out-of-body experiences, as it projects out of the physical body and flies through the astral dimension. A similar experience occurs during a near-death occurrence.

An analogy to the astral body can be made using the infrared frequency of light. Like infrared light, the astral body is heavy, sticky, slow to change. If you take an infrared picture of a chair where someone was previously sitting, even as much as two hours earlier, you can see remnants of their energy still clinging to it. Or, consider the psychic who can take a piece of clothing of a lost child and "tune in" to that being; it is through the infrared-like qualities of the child's astral energy that the psychic is able to do so.

Because of this slow, sticky quality of the astral, the emotional body acts as a magnet for experiences to stick to us, to attach themselves to the fabric of the astral body. If we hold the karmic theme of being a victim, for example, the unique vibratory quality of that "thoughtform" (a manifestation of a strong thought or emotion as an actual energetic structure within an individual's auric field) attracts situations to perpetuate the victim theme. Sometimes that energy is so obvious within a person's aura that it is as if he or she is subconsciously putting out the message, "I'm a victim — please come victimize me." Or perhaps it's not even subconscious but rather like wearing a sign on one's back that says, "Please hit me."

No matter what karmic theme is vibrating within the emotional body (fear, sadness, anger, etc.), it will perpetuate itself until we learn its lesson. The emotional body is just like the teacher who keeps giving homework assignments until the student understands the lesson. The Higher Self never lets us take a shortcut — we only release the theme when we have mastered it, and that means having looked at it from every perspective. We have to come full circle.

Four

The
Inner World
of Consciousness

*From pure joy
Springs all creation.
By joy it is sustained,
Towards joy it proceeds
And to joy it returns.*

SANSKRIT

We are each searching for our conscious connection with God, the infinite Self that holds the answers to all the questions that relate to life. But where to begin the spiritual search is a common question. In fact, the spiritual search really began a long time ago. What we need now is to make that search conscious. So once again the answer is to expand our consciousness.

Most spiritual guides would agree that meditation is essential to that expansion. If you haven't learned to meditate, do so. If you have learned a technique with which you are happy, then meditate regularly. There are many techniques of meditation. For one to be useful, it does not have to be difficult. I prefer the Transcendental Meditation (TM) technique because it is based on effortlessness. The more simple and natural something is, usually the more powerful it is. This is true for TM. It is a technique that takes the attention inward to increasingly refined, more silent levels of awareness until the person arrives at the simplest level of awareness, silence, and then transcends into pure consciousness: a field of no thought, no activity — just unbounded silence. This impersonal God-consciousness, as it is called, is the source of thinking — the All, Absolute, Nonchanging, Eternal, Infinite. From this source of nature, anything can be manifested. It is said that enlightenment can be attained when this pure being, or pure consciousness, is maintained on the level of consciousness, 24 hours a day. This is the realization of the Self.

Meditation should be a comfortable, enjoyable experience. It is not time for "internal work" — that should be done separately. It is a time of transcendence, a time to be with the Self. Therefore, it is a rejuvenating, awakening time period. It is a preparation for activity, and its purpose is to bring more awareness and more of our potential into our moment-to-moment living.

At the Deva Foundation we use a different process. Whereas meditation is passive and designed to just *be*, to transcend thought and shift into the silence, the Deva sessions are mentally active and emotional. They are designed to perform action from the depths of pure being and bring the guidance and wisdom of that field of all possibilities into conscious life, using the Higher Self as the interpreter. Both processes are important to our transformational work. Therefore, we suggest a daily schedule of meditation plus Deva sessions every few months as a powerful combination for growth, one that will complement any other inner processing a person may be doing.

The TM technique involves an "inward stroke" and an "outward stroke." The inward stroke expands consciousness by taking us deep inside, breaking boundaries of limitation and constriction. To learn the inward stroke is to learn to go within. Once you become familiar with this process and familiar with the subtle levels of thought, you will move your evolution forward exponentially. If someone asked me the single most-important step toward enlightenment, I would say, "Learn to go within the Self. Learn to transcend the superficial levels of life."

The outward stroke creates an energetic clearing of the limitations to pure consciousness. It has the effect of releasing stress, whether physical or emotional, and harmonizing the energy flow. By releasing the energetic blockages, we find holistic change in our life, which fact is documented by hundreds of scientific studies on the benefits of TM.

Symbolically, the outward stroke also implies using a clearer perception and efficiency of thinking to take dynamic action in our world, to live life based on the platform of pure consciousness. In this way, we fulfill desire by manifesting our infinite potential from that platform.

The inward stroke, then, takes us to our God source and saturates us with clarity and peacefulness, while the outer stroke clears the mental and emotional "static" out as well as making it possible to radiate our light into life.

Once a person has learned to go within, a new world opens. There are many techniques for mental prowess and manifesta-tion, but the ability to entertain thought on deeper and more powerful levels of awareness is the key to success. Anything is possible on the level of pure consciousness, for the simple reason that pure consciousness is God, though purely abstract. Therefore, it truly is a field of pure potential waiting to be drawn into form. The degree of fulfillment we experience in life is dependent on the degree of stabilization of this "home" of all the laws of nature and our ability to use that potential in living.

For example, if a person wants an apple, it is necessary to take action to fulfill that desire. Depending on how powerful and clear the consciousness is, there may be a differing degree of effort and time lapse between the moment of the desire and its fulfillment. A person experiencing only a small portion of his or her potential, for example, may have to get in the car and drive to several markets before finding the right apple. That exertion may be stressful to the point that the taste of the apple may be diminished or overshadowed by the difficulty of the task of finding it.

If a person is a little more conscious, however, then he or she may walk out to the car to start the search but perhaps immediately notices an apple stand across the street that sells big, juicy apples. The delight at such a "synchronicity" adds to the enjoyment of the apple.

As a person becomes even more conscious, the ability to manifest the desire increases. This time, for example, the person has the thought about the apple, and instantly there is a knock at the door from a friend who has stopped by with a gift of eight delicious apples! Again, the effortlessness and speed of the process have increased to further the fulfillment.

One more step toward effortlessness would be the ability to have the desire and then manifest the apple in the hand — like Jesus changing water into wine, or any other miracle of consciousness. Pure mastery of the laws of nature provide one more step to perfect efficiency. At the same moment as we have the thought, which is coming from the source of "all possibility" within us, we can have immediate gratification of that desire on the level of consciousness. The apple is tasted, the nourishment is felt, and the fulfillment is complete — instantly. There is no time delay, no struggle — just the bliss of pure being.

As our potential holistically evolves, we will find that life becomes easier, and we will live it with less struggle and more immediate fulfillment. This state of enlightenment is the birthright of every individual. The secret lies within!

(As I was writing this analogy of the apple, a beautiful confirmation experience occurred. Earlier that morning Paula and I had been talking about our desire for some chicken tamales sold only on Saturdays from a small Hispanic kitchen twenty miles away in Santa Fe. But because of our busy schedule there was not time to drive into town, so we put the desire out of our minds.

An hour later, our friends Mike and Marian Martinez came to the house with several bags of chicken tamales. I was so excited about the synchronicity of this event that I read them the apple analogy. Mike said, "You should put me in the book!" So, here it is, Mike!)

As our ability to inwardly transcend develops, we have access to an expanded world of information and knowledge. Every level within us holds a different state of consciousness, a new reality that is rich in its knowledge. A simple example is dream interpretation, where we can use the information gained in the dream state to better understand ourselves in our waking state of consciousness.

The purpose of knowledge is to develop skill in action. Through knowledge we gain understanding, and we use that understanding to grow, to change, to move from a limited emotional reaction (like anger) to a more flowing response (like compassion). As we use knowledge to move through a change, the world around us changes — our point of view has been altered. This process can be likened to climbing a tree. By taking a step up to a higher branch, we can see from a different perspective. Now we are ready to gain more knowledge in order to take the next step up the tree of knowledge. But we can become attached to a particular form of knowledge as easily as we become attached to anger. Unless we use knowledge and then go beyond it to even more expansive knowledge, we will be stuck on a single branch of the tree.

Knowledge is relative. What I have found to be "true" for myself may be inappropriate for someone else. The only absolute knowledge is that which is unchanging and eternal, the pure knowledge of God-consciousness. If we continue to use knowledge and understanding without attachment, one day we will arrive at the top of the tree and experience the unbounded Self. Then we will no longer need the tree of knowledge. We can jump into being and just radiate its essence. But to reach the wisdom of God, we must first become conscious that we are looking for the Divinity, and we must be awake on the path. As life carries us forward through many different external experiences, we must be moving inwardly also, deeper and deeper.

Our visible life is an expression of the choices we have made on a soul level in order to understand our remaining karmic lessons. The physical body is one external manifestation of the themes of the emotional body. The situations we find ourselves moving through are the "stages" we create in order to have a theater in which to play out our roles, to enact the drama of *being in relationship*. There is a lot to learn about ourselves by looking at our patterns and acknowledging the feelings that are triggered in the tangible world around us. This is where knowledge and understanding on the inner levels can help to change our lives. But we will never fully understand ourselves without also looking at the inner dimensions. Carl Gustav Jung called that inner world the subconscious, the realm of symbols and abstraction. To enter this world without confusion, we need to learn a new language and follow new rules of thinking and feeling.

When clients arrive to do sessions at the Deva Foundation, one of the first steps in the process is to expand their understanding of symbols and their ability to work on that level. If people have already accomplished this, then they are ready to use their knowledge to move deeply within their astral nature. If not, the Deva facilitator will help them begin to understand the language of symbols and how it relates to their life. Symbols are the language of the astral and spiritual dimensions.

Anytime we go within to do inner work, meditate, or dream, symbols can be the keys to profound understanding. They translate the content of the subconscious mind to us and can be interpreted on many levels. For example, consider the symbol of the white dove. White can be equated with purity (a blending of all the colors of the rainbow); dove can be viewed as a prophetic bird that can fly free (the bird of peace, gentleness, and love).

Therefore, so the symbol may represent that which is essential and authentic within us.

Depending on the context in which the symbol appears, we then use this symbol as a key to unlock the understanding it has to offer us. Does the white dove come at a time of panic, struggle, or conflict? If so, it may be the energy of peace and gentleness to calm our restlessness or the sign that shows us that peace is the solution to our worries and that we should take action to find that peace. Or the white dove may simply be a sign of confirmation that helps us to trust our actions. I find that many people may not intellectually understand the meaning of a symbol — or even care to — but that the symbol still produces an effect that brings some abstract knowing on a deep level and very often a smile of acknowledgment to the face.

After a person has started to pay attention to the inner world of symbols, he or she begins to be aware of the connection to the outer world, to daily life. This new way of "seeing" is both a bridging of the inner and outer points of view and an indication of our ability to stay in tune with the Higher Self, as it brings us messages through the use of symbols. Our awareness expands when we open to another source of information. If we look at a photograph of a white dove and then glance out the window to see a white dove flying by, we might have several possible reactions. From the "objective" point of view of the scientist, this event would likely be seen as chance or coincidence. To someone else it might be seen as an amusing oddity. But if we are open to symbolic meaning, it can produce a profound shift of energy that could change our lives.

Symbols are the language of the Higher Self because symbols are energy, and they are, by definition, multidimensional. At the heart of a karmic theme there is a symbol that holds the hologram of that lesson. Since the symbol is energy, it has a unique frequency that is common to everyone. By observing other people working through their experiences of emotional or karmic themes, we can learn about ourselves. We each experience the symbolic emotional themes in our own individual way and from our unique point of view, but the symbol itself is universal, as is its vibrational energy. The emotional body holds the spectrum of possibilities that we choose to experience until we have become free from our attachment to our karmic themes. As a result, we can then integrate the many vibrations of karma into a oneness like the rainbow. And like the rainbow, the karmic lessons are visible but not binding, an inspiration to life.

The client's Higher Self takes her or him into the symbolic energies of various emotional themes. These energies may manifest to consciousness as a story the Higher Self creates to expose the theme that is of the greatest importance to the individual's development at that particular moment. If, for example, a person is sick with a sore throat, the Higher Self will probably take her or him to the source of the emotional theme that is responsible for creating that illness. This process may take the form of a purely symbolic story about not speaking one's truth or, possibly, about the suppression of strong judgmental feelings — there are many possibilities. The experience the Higher Self reveals will always bring a change of energy to the current situation.

Alternatively, the Higher Self might take the attention to one of the imprinted layers of experience that is still clinging to astral memory. This is another way of saying that we must "peel the onion" of a particular emotional issue, which has been created over time and contains many layers of related emotional experiences. If I am concerned with the issue of self-judgment, for example, I surely have experienced countless incidences where the self-judgment theme has been repeated, though probably each situation is slightly different. Each time this occurs, another layer is produced on top of the previous layer of memory in the emotional body, and the onion grows. It is very difficult to remove the entire onion at once, so the Higher Self begins the healing by peeling one layer — or sometimes several — at a time, until eventually the core of the emotional theme is exposed and then energetically released.

It is not important to distinguish between the Higher Self's symbolic fabrication of a story and an actual memory of the past, because from the perspective of the emotional body, both are lived as a reality, as "truth." Most of the time the client intuitively just "knows" the difference between a symbol or metaphor and an actual past-life memory.

As the client begins to experience the spiritual perspective revealed by the story or past-life vignette, the Higher Self expands our understanding of the theme, or at the very least stimulates a process of energy transmutation to resolve the theme. In order to change any system of thought — or system of nature — there must be an input of energy. The emotional body will repeat endlessly a karmic theme until action is taken to change the pattern.

The action we take at the Deva Foundation is to access the energy and perspective of the Higher Self, which always knows why we have chosen a particular lesson and, more importantly, what action to take to bring it to resolution. An analogy can be made to computer programming. Let's say we have been using an old "computer program" of the emotional body that is outdated and obsolete. The mind body is skilled at running the program, but it does not have the expertise to reprogram the computer with new, appropriate software programs. So we make the choice to bring in the expert. The Higher Self not only knows how to reprogram the computer, it knows the perfect program we need at that moment. By accessing the expert, we save time and energy, thus producing greater efficiency of action.

The sessions at the Deva Foundation, like meditation, consist of an inward and an outward stroke of consciousness. The inward stroke is representative of the yin energy, which involves moving deep into the divine nature and contacting the Higher Self, the divine knowing within each person. By cultivating the inward stroke, we access the guidance we need to learn our lessons. The Higher Self then takes us into our karmic themes in the most efficient way possible for us at that moment, helping us to energetically transform limitation into freedom, ignorance into knowledge.

The outward stroke of change, purification, and transformation is one of action, an expression of the yang energy. The outward stroke is at times unpleasant. It can be intensely emotional, startling, and even physically stressful, but at the same time, we understand that the emotional residue is exiting from inside of us, which results in a feeling of release and a knowledge that life will be pleasantly different. There may be resistance to facing the repressed memories inside, but once a person moves through just one clearing session in which he or she has confronted the "unspeakable," the fear disappears and is replaced by an optimism for living, even an attitude of "bring me more — I can handle anything!" It can be very inspirational to watch, this mastering of the inward and outward strokes of our evolutionary process.

It is important to understand how these memories energetically attach to the emotional body. We must remember that we are a collection of subtle bodies, all existing within us on different vibratory octaves. Since the emotional body exists in negative space-time, it has a magnetic characteristic. This magnetic effect attracts thoughtforms and locks them into its energetic "groove," like an enzyme locking onto a protein molecule. The result of this attraction-connection interplay is the experience of the emotion and the "feeding" of that energy into the emotional body. This is not much different from the physical body requiring food to perpetuate itself, which it will therefore seek, sometimes with obsession. The question of where this initial "groove" comes from will be discussed in chapter 8.

The following simple model encapsulates this process: "If I own the emotional thoughtform of (_____), I create/attract (_____) in my surroundings." We can fill in the blank with any emotional theme; theoretically, it can be positive or negative. It can be happiness or sadness, peace or anger, love or hate. Most commonly, given an emotional body full of karmic attachments, we see the creation/attraction of what is perceived as a negative emotional theme, but inherent within it is the opportunity for resolution and subsequent expansion. However, as we often see, this model can also repeat itself ad infinitum. For example, if I hold the theme of rejection within my emotional body, this thoughtform will magnetically create/attract an experience of rejection in my surroundings. As the process is set in motion, I will witness myself attracting an actor to play the role of victimizer, as I repeat the role of the victim of rejection. For at the same time as I play the victim of this theme, there is always someone out there with the complementary karmic theme of victimizer, who will eagerly play that role. But while it is important to see what polarity of victim-victimizer we choose, the theme is essentially the same. In this case, it is the rejection theme with its particular magnetic astral signature that creates/attracts other astral signatures that match, so that we can enact the drama one more time.

In addition to this individual creation/attraction process, it is conceivable that these thoughtforms can exist independently. Says Dr. Richard Gerber, "The astral domain has certain unique properties, one of which is that astrally or emotionally charged thoughts have a life of their own. At the astral energetic level, certain thoughts, either conscious or unconscious, may exist as distinct energy fields or thoughtforms with unique shapes, colors, and characteristics. Some thoughts, especially those that are charged with emotional intensity, can have a separate identity apart from their creator. Certain thoughts may actually be charged with subtle energetic substance and exist (unconsciously) as thoughtforms in the energetic fields of their creators. Those thoughtforms can frequently be seen by clairvoyant individuals who are very sensitive to higher energetic phenomena" (*Vibrational Medicine*, p. 151).

Besides clearing the magnetically attached aspects of the emotional body, we need to clear the clinging, negative thoughtforms from the collective consciousness of this planet and beyond. The implication is that even though I may have resolved my attachment to certain thoughtforms — hate, for example — and have erased their ability to attach to my emotional body, those thoughtforms still exist. I may have responsibility toward their creation from the past, and therefore I have responsibility for neutralizing them with my love in the present. This is another demonstration of the fact that we are not separate, that we affect everyone and everything in the universe, and that we have a responsibility to help purify the collective consciousness.

It is not uncommon during sessions for the person to have an experience of seeing, resolving, and releasing these universal themes with the distinct knowing that they are working on a global level and not just individually. The added benefit is that there is always a realization of greater "unity consciousness" growing within them. Experience tells me that more and more people are breaking the constraints of personal limitation and, as a result, they are free to extend their efforts to a more universal scale.

Today we hear a lot about the concept of positive thinking and the use of affirmations. The theory is that by bringing our attention to a spiritual virtue, such as "I'm happy," we focus the mind on its desire, thus setting in motion the process of, in this case, creating happiness. However, just thinking or saying "I'm happy, I'm happy . . . " does not by itself release the themes of unhappiness, sadness, disappointment, and so forth from the emotional body. The proper intention can move the cloud away from the sun for a while, perhaps, but the cloud still exists. We must go much deeper and get at the root of the problem before we can resolve it.

So while making the choice to turn toward positivity is important, it is just as important to acknowledge the negative. It is interesting that when we say "the negative," we are making a judgment of good and bad. Why should we feel that our karma or emotional-body themes are bad? I prefer to see the "negative" emotional-body themes as our *opportunities* for learning, for becoming wiser and more loving. The "positive" can be seen as the spiritual virtues of life expressing through enlightened awareness: by directing our attention to the sun, it will give us strength to more efficiently dissolve the clouds that overshadow it. Therefore the perfect formula is *awareness of both*, the cloud and the sun; this way we can see the big picture without denial or repression.

It is common these days with New Age groups to try to shut out the "negative," to try to insulate oneself "in the light." However, to withdraw from any aspect of the world is to separate oneself still further from unity. When a person reaches unity consciousness, does he or she feel unified only with the pure mountain stream and not the polluted pond? Does not the enlightened person acknowledge the suffering of others? We may no longer need to choose suffering, but we must be aware of it. We are not separate!

In Chinese and other philosophies, there is a precept that the microcosm mirrors the macrocosm — that all is one and the laws that apply on a universal scale also apply to the individual. If there is suffering in the world, then there is a dimension of my being that is suffering. If there is a boy starving in Africa, part of me is starving. To deny the situation of the boy is to deny an aspect of my being. I may not have the means to physically save the boy, but I have the means on the level of awareness to have understanding and compassion, to radiate love. Through the coherence of love's energy comes a subtle — sometimes tangible — stimulation of that frequency of karma within myself that can heal individually and collectively the world's symbolic starvation. If I have cleared my individual emotional body's theme of starvation, then by bringing awareness to the boy, I have an opportunity to take a further step. Whatever the situation, however, awareness is mandatory. The more awareness we have, the more powerful our social actions will be. Action always follows from awareness. As our awareness grows, our ability to change the world is magnified.

Through the news of the famine in Africa in the late 1980s, a tremendous wave of love and support, both spiritually and materially, was generated. Not only were many lives saved, but an attitude of hope and altruism was fostered in those people who took action and saw the benefit of that action. One hundred years ago we may not have known what was happening to our African neighbors, and thus we would not have reached out to help. A benefit of our technological age is that we can be more aware on a global level and take global action.

Five

The Chakras &
Emotional-Body
Dynamics

*When we let go of the resistance,
we penetrate to the direct
experience of the distraction,
and its quality of distractedness,
its discomfort, dissolves
in the clear seeing of it.*

STEPHEN LEVINE
A Gradual Awakening

*T*here is a direct relationship
between consciousness and the physical nervous system. We can
say that consciousness expresses itself through the nerve pathways
and the functioning of the brain. One expression of consciousness
is seen in the relative degree of wakefulness and alertness. For
example, when we sleep poorly in the night, the next day seems
to be a struggle because tiredness and foggy perception have overshadowed our awareness. Alternatively, a good night's sleep brings
greater alertness to the mind and more calmness to the body. And
when there is greater restfulness and wakefulness in the mind and
body, our receptivity to the world inside of us and around us

61

is enhanced. Therefore, the consciousness that expresses through us is dependent on the condition and function of the nervous system but also of all the subtle bodies.

As we look closely at people in our lives, we are able to witness the different compositions and expressions of their emotional bodies. To the emotional body, energy is energy. The more it feeds, the hungrier it gets, just like the drug addict. In fact, as we look deep into the dynamics of how the emotional body functions, it becomes clearer that one characteristic can be described as "the addict."

The addictions of the emotional body exist because of an underlying desire for pleasure, for expansion, and, ultimately, for unity with God. This desire is fundamental because it is the evolutionary force that genetically pushes us forward to the knowledge and experience of God/Infinity/Bliss. This experience is potentially available to each of us on the level of pure consciousness, that fundamental essence of life. Our deepest memories are calling us back to the source of our consciousness, and we yearn to experience it permanently.

The subtle bodies are always interfacing and affecting the physical body, especially the nervous system. As the energy flows from the physical body through the etheric body into the realm of the subtle bodies and back, this energy stimulates our being in countless ways. For example, in those places of the emotional body where we are holding a karmic attachment, such as anger, the passing energy will stimulate this place of attachment, creating a reaction such as subconscious anger; this may then be repressed or expressed outwardly. Either way, the anger has been triggered, and a reaction (stimulus) occurs. This activity may accumulate and become quite intense physically or emotionally, and it may produce chaos and disorder in the functioning of the nervous system due to the energetic blockages. Our consciousness is adversely affected by this energy flow.

The subtle bodies and the physical body are also affected by the external environment. The senses open the flow of energy from the environment into our consciousness and that stimuli interacts with our internal programming. For example, watching a horror movie can trigger issues of fear in the emotional body. The effect of the sum total of all the internal and external stimuli on our consciousness is measured by what is called the "arousal level."

A balance between yin and yang energies creates an optimum arousal level, where there are no overshadowing influences resulting from too much or too little of either. This optimum level is desirable because it provides us with a baseline level of enjoyment that is lasting, stable, and fulfilling. Those moments when the mind is calm and clear and the body is rested and relaxed, with a feeling of peace radiating through the internal and external environments, are a sign of an optimum arousal level.

Our arousal level fluctuates in a range moving higher and lower depending on what is happening both outside of us and within us and the degree of consciousness that is manifesting through us in the form of alertness and wakefulness. If the arousal level goes up, then the sum total of stimuli moving through us has increased, or our ability to process the stimulation has been faulty or inefficient, and we are left with an accumulation of energy, like water behind a dam. If the arousal level goes down from that high level, then the stimulus has been reduced, or our ability to process it has become more efficient, and the effect is like a calmly flowing river.

If the arousal level goes down from this balanced baseline level, we feel an imbalance of yin energy, resulting in boredom and depressive feelings. The energy flow becomes deficient, and the emotional body either becomes attached and feeds on the weakness syndrome or will create/attract "victim" themes to stimulate the emotional excitement of tragedy. This, of course, may temporarily pull the arousal level up.

If the arousal level goes up above optimum, then the yang energy creates excitement. In the nervous system, the sympathetic nervous system will be triggered, resulting in the reaction that is commonly referred to as the "fight-flight response." This excitation expends energy, boosting the metabolism; it stimulates adrenaline secretion into the bloodstream, causing the heart rate to go up, with other tension-producing effects. This excitement can produce a sensation of pleasure, but it is usually short-lived, the variable being the duration of the stimulus and/or the ability of the nervous system to process the stimuli.

If the excitement brings pleasure, then the desire for more pleasure is always triggered. As this excitement response is repeated, habituation sets in, that phenomenon of familiarity to a recurring experience that lessens the excitement and pleasure. As we become habituated to a given level of excitation, we need more stimulus to receive the same subjective degree of pleasure.

Drug addiction is the obvious example. Relative to the arousal level, an addict has become habituated to a high level of excitement and in daily life will feel bored and a compelling need for more excitement, more pleasure. So the person will take more drugs to reach a "high." But habituation knows no limit, and the addict will self-destruct while striving for the ever-elusive state of bliss.

On the emotional-body level, we can see the sticky, astral nature of the emotional body as the addict. Not only does it need stimulus to provide energy to feed on in order to survive, but it also knows no limit. It doesn't care whether what it attracts is pleasurable or painful. There may be brief moments of satiety in the beginning stages, but it will then set the stage to create/attract more stimulus on which to feed itself. We can call it karmic repetition or we can call it "sabotage," but the impetus for the emotional-body cravings is the same as for all our dimensions of self: the desire for unity with the source of love, God.

The problem is that if we attempt to find satiation and fulfillment in an outer direction, in the "material world," the result will always be temporary and eventually incomplete. There will always be something new to buy, some new pleasure to seek. But if we direct our attention inward, bringing conscious awareness to the spiritual dimensions, that transcendental world of the infinite Self, we will instead satiate ourselves with the highest vibratory energies. This activity balances the arousal level, and this balance of yin and yang produces the ability for enjoyment. As a result, our daily baseline arousal level is open and receptive to diversity within the unity, activity within the silence, and feelings with love as their basis.

For most of us, our arousal level has been raised above the optimum level because we do not take the time to balance our energies through spiritual practice or the benefit of spiritual experience. We may not exhibit serious addictions, but just having our attention primarily directed externally to our outer life will eventually pull us further out of balance. As we get caught up in the excitement/habituation vicious cycle, more and more energy is directed outwardly and into securing our astral attachments to the emotional body, like an addict looking for a drug.

Besides the draining effect physically, there is also an imprinting process that's happening physically. The karmic patterns, thoughtforms, and so on are not only imprinted in the emotional body but also etherically, and the etheric imprints then act as templates to imprint the physical body. For example, if a person smokes ten cigarettes per day, the nicotine (which is one of the most addicting substances on the planet) and other chemicals in the cigarette create a physiological stress on the body initially, causing it to react defensively to the invasion of the "smoke." Quickly, however, the cigarette's influence overshadows the physical body's reaction, and it astrally attaches itself to the emotional body, causing the beginning of the addiction and habituation process.

Emotionally, there may be numerous reasons to choose to smoke. One of the most common is to effectively close the door on the feelings of sadness, loneliness, and isolation that are usually held in the lungs. As the smoke paralyzes the ch'i of the lungs, it also paralyzes that life energy that would help us to expose and look closely at our emotional themes that are held in the lungs, themes that were probably already in existence within us before we chose to smoke. This is an example of how karma from past lives can be the explanation for why we choose such things in today's life. Perhaps the sadness has created a vulnerability that then leaves us open to seduction by such things as smoking or other addictions.

The reality is that we are sabotaging ourselves, becoming the victims of our habits, and if these addictions are left unchecked, we are making a choice for slow death. Make no mistake of denial here. To choose to smoke is to choose to slowly kill yourself. The intellect may understand the risk, but its wisdom may be overshadowed by the emotional body's use of the addiction to control the situation and perpetuate itself.

For us to free ourselves from these addictive patterns, there must be an inward stroke to direct our attention to the Self, to unbounded awareness, to silence. This meditative process will help lower our hyper-arousal level or raise our hypo-arousal level into the optimum state of being.

A person undergoing detoxification from chemical abuse goes through massive chemical changes in the physical body, but it is the underlying astral "detoxification" that is really producing the physical pain and emotional trauma. We seem to be concerned about the temporary insanity that results when a person is detoxifying, but we fail to see the insanity of people's lives while the "astral drug" is alive and well within them. Again, our individual view of reality is dependent on the boundaries of our consciousness.

Because the subtle bodies coexist with the physical body, we can hold emotional imprints anywhere within the physical body: a feeling of being "heartbroken" over the loss of a loved one can be held in the heart; a feeling of powerlessness over losing a job or a mate can be held in the arms or back; even a memory of having our head chopped off in a past life can leave an imprint in the neck. Over the years I have watched myself and hundreds of others release energy from every possible part of the physical body.

The emotional body is also intelligent, and its voice is what I call the ego. The ego is identified with its "body" and therefore the karmic themes that are attached to it. The expression of the ego is the expression of the emotional body. When the emotional body speaks, for example through feelings of helplessness, sadness, and so on, the ego expresses its identification with those feelings by being helpless and sad; it knows no other reality until the next feeling arrives. The ego speaks in its unique voice from the gut, specifically the solar plexus chakra. All of its karmic attachments, which are structured multidimensionally through the various subtle bodies, reflex to the solar plexus. This chakra is therefore unique, because all emotional themes have an effect in this chakra.

This may be the reason why there is so much controversy about which chakra controls which emotion. For example, power is an issue for most people; the state of our planet mirrors this fact to us dramatically. There are those who believe that power is controlled by the solar plexus chakra. Since the solar plexus is the seat of the emotional body and a control center for all of the emotional themes, it is common that the many expressions of the abuse of power or the loss of power would be seen as being held in this chakra. But power has many manifestations, and one can see its expression in almost every chakra. The crown chakra and "third eye" (the area directly behind the center of the forehead) certainly express a spiritual power. The heart chakra expresses the infinite power of love. As we move into the chakras below the heart area, we begin to see the expression of the attachments to power.

I personally believe that our issues with power are held at the source of our energy, the first chakra. The red energy of the first chakra is fundamental to our life, just as power is fundamental to taking action of any kind. I don't feel that power opens into expression later in our evolution, which would be symbolized by it being structured within the solar plexus, but rather that power has been structured within our being since the beginning of our incarnations. We are born from the infinite power of God, and we "go home" to that infinite power when we physically die. Through the first chakra we are born, and it is that power of creation that lies at the source of life, symbolized by the first chakra.

Because of the many interrelationships of our personal experiences and therefore our karmic attachments, the expression of these emotional themes within the chakras can be complex and sometimes unfathomable. If we take the idea that emotion is energy with a unique vibratory rate that is expressed as color, then the "color" of anger will be different from the "color" of fear. Because these two emotions are quite different energies, they are not expressed simultaneously, but rather one gives rise to the other: fear becomes anger. On the physical level, the dirty yellow of fear or its energetic companion cowardice (cowards have traditionally been dubbed "yellow") can be seen transforming into the yang dirty red of anger ("red with anger"). In the transition there may be a moment of orange (yellow plus red creates orange).

However, the distinctions are not always so clear-cut. Seduction, for example, can be a misuse of sexual power, having its characteristic color, and manipulation can be a misuse of emotional or mental power, with its corresponding shade; however, if both are operating simultaneously, the energies can mix into a reddish-greenish brown color in which it is difficult to see energetically what is being felt. Or if a person is dealing with a past-life memory in which all these energies are imprinted together and, in addition, the current life feelings are impinging upon and combining with its release, an aura reader or clairvoyant may easily misinterpret what is happening emotionally.

While it is true that the rays of the chakras can be a blueprint for our karmic themes, even the clearest psychic reader can make mistakes. Therefore, it is essential that we each develop our own inner knowing and use it to discover the mysteries within and around us — that we use self-knowledge to understand ourselves. One way this happens is through the process of inner work guided by the Higher Self.

A theme that most everyone today is working on is the abuse or misuse of sexual energy. I have yet to have a client who didn't have some stress or residue from sexual experience or the various programming experienced growing up, especially in the West. Sexual karma is seldom isolated in our experience — it often is associated with such yang energies as power, control, domination, manipulation, and seduction. What these words have in common is their source in the energy field of the first chakra and their addicting influence on the seat to the emotional body, the solar plexus.

The first or "root" chakra is located in the perineum, near the base of the spine. It is the source of our life force, the basic energy that moves up through the body. Its vibration is red, the slowest frequency but the most abundant and commonly the most powerful energy we radiate, as can be seen by the above examples.

The easiest way to understand the function and purpose of the root chakra is to comprehend its fundamental survival needs: food, oxygen, water, shelter/protection, and procreation. In order to obtain food and water, the primitive "cave man" within us will use his red energy regardless of the situation. If he is hungry enough, he will use his power to fight to fulfill his needs. So the aggressive masculine themes of misuse of power, hate, anger, violence, and so forth create a major imprint in the emotional body. These themes are very energetic — sometimes subconsciously we experience someone's hate or anger, for example, as if they are hurling a ball of red energy at us — and we've learned well how to put up our defenses to protect ourselves.

This defensive reaction is initiated by the emotional body and is often seen as the closing of the solar plexus chakra, but the need for protection actually originates in the first chakra. The most obvious example is our general auric field, that buffer zone to the environment around us. It's important to understand that this aura is made of mostly yang energy; the Chinese doctor calls it *wei ch'i*, that which keeps the "pernicious evils" out and keeps our immune system strong and resistant to outside influences. The strength of our personal "shelter/protection" system depends on the vitality and flow of our first-chakra system. Of all the chakras, the advice to "keep the energy moving" is most important for the first chakra, because it provides core energy to the rest of the chakras and to the body as a whole. Low-energy problems usually originate in the imbalance or blockage of the first chakra.

Another key survival need is the genetic demand for procreation. At this point in history, procreation is not much of a concern due to overpopulation; however, the sexual drive is an issue for almost everyone. The sexual need is strong for many reasons, but the least obvious is that it comes from the same energetic source as our power and other masculine themes, the first chakra. From my experience, a person who has a strong first-chakra energy also has a strong sexual drive. This drive may not be obvious, however, because he or she may channel that sexual energy in other creative ways.

What happens when the sexual energy becomes associated with the negative masculine themes of the first chakra? The answer provides the beginning of our understanding of why there is so much first-chakra karma and, consequently, why there is so much debate and controversy about the three-letter word *sex*. The story in chapter 6 of a Swedish man named Olaf provides a good example of these issues.

The emotional body is an addict. The stimulus arising from the first chakra is usually unparalleled by any of the other chakras, probably due to its powerful energetic nature. The "hit" of hate, anger, or violence is very addicting, just like the "hit" of orgasm. This may be why some religions have condemned "sex for pleasure." When the sexual energy gets muddied by any of the negative masculine themes, such as hate or violence, then the classic case of rape results. Whether one is the victim or victimizer of the rape experience, the emotional body will imprint that memory, and being the addict that it is, it will crave more and more and more. Here we have the repetition of karma through many lifetimes. Because the sexual energy is so powerful, it is also a potentially dangerous addiction for the emotional body.

This point of view may be in contrast with the fundamentalist religious point of view that the sexual energy may be dangerous to the soul and, therefore, to *all areas* of our life. Dogma is then deemed necessary to protect the individual and society. The dogma is usually understood to mean "sex is for procreation only," "sex is not for pleasure," or "sex is not for spiritual evolution." In addition, we have passed down through the generations the programming that to be holy and pure is to be celibate. Wasn't Jesus celibate? Aren't all the monks and priests celibate? Therefore, to be chaste is to be spiritual. Of course, there have been a few exceptions, like Krishna and Buddha, who taught so much about sexual love and who also evolved through sexual experience, but their examples have usually been overshadowed in the West by the Christian ethic.

It is time to clear away the confusion and ignorance around sexuality. The challenge for us now is to accept our sexuality as a fundamental part of being human, but also to acknowledge that there are many sexual imprints — and even more first-chakra imprints — in the emotional body to resolve and learn from. To bring awareness into the first chakra is to begin the balancing of core energy. Then we can use the clear power of the first chakra to literally perform miracles in our lives.

In 1977, I had my first taste of the power of the first-chakra energy. Maharishi Mahesh Yogi was teaching me and others Patanjali's *yoga sutra* meditation technique for levitation. The first meditation was enough to send me into the air with a shout. I expected to gracefully lift into the air like a butterfly, but the experience more closely approximated being propelled into the sky like a rocket blasting off! The energy started at the base of my spine and shot through me, literally sending me flying in one big hop. I began to understand that when we clear the blockages in our lower chakras, the unlimited potential of these chakras will unfold in ways that make the word "miracle" obsolete.

My levitation experiences have always felt "sexual" in the sense that the sexual energy filled my body. As a result, sexual experience has always felt very much like an aspect of a Kundalini experience; in fact, it is the same energy. It is time to be free to know it and use it for our personal evolution.

Six

A Case Study of Sexual Karma

*The Higher Self wants to tell me
that you can use all the
sexual energy you want, but
it must be used from a point
of love, understanding,
and enlightenment.*

OLAF

A good example of how a person can bring awareness to his or her first-chakra karmic/emotional themes is given by the experience of a man named Olaf, who is from Sweden. This 50-year-old man became conscious of his first-chakra addictions — seduction, manipulation, abuse of power, survival, sexual compulsive behavior, and promiscuity — and did a session to try to find greater understanding and release the addictions. The following account is a word-for-word transcription of his session. (The bracketed material represents the observations of the facilitator.)

The facilitator asked Olaf to climb up onto the massage table, close his eyes, and rest for a few minutes. Then the facilitator stimulated the appropriate acupuncture points (through various massage techniques) and with the help of breathing techniques slowly guided Olaf inward with a white-light meditation exercise, allowing his consciousness to open and his energy to quicken in vibration. His Higher Self was then asked to come in and make contact. With that channel open to his divine inner knowing, Olaf was ready to work.

Facilitator: *Ask your Higher Self to take you into a lifetime or experience held in your first chakra that needs to be seen and released today.*

Olaf: I'm lying on a couch. I look Roman; I'm wearing silk; there's music, food, and wine. There are a lot of girls around me; they all serve me, dance around me, touch me, and fondle me. I respond to their fondling.

It's a big villa, overlooking the sea. I have a great fortune. I just enjoy myself. I look similar to how I look today, but with more weight — similar head shape and limbs. I used to be a warrior, high up in the hierarchy, stationed in the Middle East region. I became rich from the spoils of war. There are precious stones, etc. I'm 38 to 40 now. I had my military career for twenty years. I bought slaves from all over — from the Germanic tribes, the Mediterranean, black girls.

Facilitator: *Ask your Higher Self to take you forward in that lifetime and see what happens.*

Olaf: I'm 50 now. I just enjoy myself. I'm a very kind master, though I get stern when I'm annoyed. My opinion is that they are lucky to be here with me instead of with some lecherous master. I am aware of having sexual knowledge; sometimes I surprise one or two of the girls in their chambers with my sexual appetite.

Sometimes they cry. A part of me asks if they are homesick; the other part denies that — what more could they have? What are they complaining about? Sometimes I have compassion; other times it annoys me and I just walk out — I don't want to see that woman anymore.

I just live for eating, drinking, and making love. I fall in love with one of the women and give her special attention. After a short while, I get bored. This is one of my patterns. Now there is pain and jealousy in the house. I just start with someone else, but I feel a little bit less enthusiastic. . . .

I'm getting older; the lifestyle doesn't satisfy me anymore. Sometimes when I see one of the girls I feel the old fire again, and I have her called to me. But I feel unfulfilled after love-making — it leaves a sadness in me. To kill that sadness, I penetrate a woman again; this goes on and on. I see how I have trapped myself in being unfulfilled. I don't know how to get out of this — the pattern is so strong I don't know how to break it.

There are glimpses of what it could be like with a particular woman. She is the only one I often call to share some time — eating, talking, going for a walk. There's no need for sex every time. But I still go back to my old pattern. . . .

I'm on my deathbed now. I'm holding a cup with wine and spice in it. I'm drinking it. Some of the girls are crying — their life might change. I have no fear, no pain. I don't feel for anyone — I think as a soldier. (I was always surrounded by death.) It is my time to go, and I pass out.

[After clearing the lifetime of the residual energies, the facilitator asked Olaf's Higher Self if there was any message or commentary concerning this past life.]

Olaf: I see a brass triangle or a pyramid. It symbolizes the good use of energy. The Higher Self wants to tell me that you can use all the sexual energy you want, but it must be used from a point of love, understanding, and enlightenment.

It's to be used for your highest good. I take this knowing into my first and second chakras.

Facilitator: *Ask your Higher Self to take you into another lifetime that you need to clear from your first chakra.*

Olaf: I'm in China. I live in the household of my lord, a powerful master over people and land. He's very strong, and very hard and cruel sometimes. He has many concubines and wives. I am a concubine. I was chosen for my abilities of sex. I can seduce and exhaust my master. He loves it very much, but when I exhaust him, he often beats me. He hits me with the back of his hand on my face until I bleed. He says I'm a witch, that I take his strength away. My crying excites him; he takes me again. I just react — I can't refuse him, but I close my vaginal muscles tightly and suck him dry. Sometimes he falls asleep, or he continues to beat me. I seem to enjoy it — to enjoy this pain, the helplessness, and the power and strength I feel when I can make him helpless. (I feel sadness, helplessness, in my body now.)

I am a manipulator. I have a definite need and craving for sex all of the time. I feel if my master doesn't have sex with me, it means he doesn't love me anymore. Therefore, he loves me even when he beats me. I need his attention, so to make love is to get his attention. He gives me a gift of jewelry; he says he wants a child with me. It makes me petrified because I can't have any children. I was raped as a young girl and can't have any.

Facilitator: *Ask your Higher Self to take you back to the time when you were raped as a young girl.*

Olaf: I see horses. A warlord sweeps down into our village. We run; I stumble. I cannot escape — there are many men. I'm only ten. I fight, but they are too strong. They take me, one man after another, until I fall unconscious. I'm bleeding a lot and torn very badly — so much pain. I feel pain in my throat and in my vaginal area, like something burning inside it. I'm so helpless and so angry — my whole body is so broken, my throat is so sore. I feel so defenseless, feeling I can't do anything. Most of the people were killed; now I have no home. I eventually end up in a whorehouse, where I meet my master at age thirteen. He buys me. I feel gratitude, but no love. I'm safe from the world outside that's been so cruel. I must keep him humored and interested. I don't want to be pushed back — I need his attention. I must be better in bed than any of his women. I don't like sex, but yet I'm addicted to it. It is my weapon and tool to survive.

[Later.] My master is dead, and I'm pushed out of the household because his wives blame me for his death. They say I'm a witch, that I took his life power. They push me into the streets; I don't know what to do. I feel fear, pain, insecurity.

I become a servant girl in a drinking place — rice wine. Simple customers come here, and everyone has the right to touch me and I can't do anything about it. But I find a way — I seduce the owner, and he takes me in as his concubine. I do the same thing to him as I did with my other master. I seduce him to have food and shelter. One day I cannot sleep with him anymore — it is disgusting. I'm abused, and I abuse myself. I want to run, but I don't know where. He forces me to have sex all of the time. I spit in his face and scratch him, kick him. He takes a fire poker and bashes my skull. I feel the pain in my forehead up to my crown. I'm lying there, but I'm not dead yet. Men come and put me on a cart and throw me into the river. I'm drowning. I'm so weak, in pain, but I also feel relief. I don't have any fear anymore. It's almost peace.

[Facilitator gives instructions for clearing the energetic memories of that past lifetime.]

Olaf: I see a sun, a rotating light coming toward me. It's spiraling like a vortex. I feel drawn to it. I disappear into that light and become one with that light. I feel great warmth, healing, and relaxation.

My Higher Self tells me to operate from that point of enlightened sexual energy. There is no longer a need to seduce to survive and be loved.

Olaf's session could be analyzed multidimensionally to the degree that another book would be necessary to comment on so many universal themes. The following commentary will focus only on the main points of his experience.

Olaf sees himself as the master, with the power to provide himself with pleasure. He has "music, food, wine, a lot of girls. . . . They all serve me . . . touch me and fondle me." He has a life in which he can indulge himself with whatever he wants, especially *bodily* wants. "I used to be a warrior. . . . I became rich from the spoils of war." The "warrior" symbolizes the first-chakra masculine themes of aggression, violence, the victimizer, and the use of power to be victorious and get rich. He has had many years of power and the imprint of being successful with it, so now he can indulge himself with its fruits.

He goes forward to age 50, which is Olaf's current age. He sees himself as the kind master, but is of the opinion that "they are lucky to be here with me instead of with some lecherous master." (His idea of "lecherous" may be debatable!) The sexual themes start to come into focus as he discusses his "sexual appetite." There is a need for control and an insensitivity to the needs of the women: "What more could they have? What are they complaining about? . . . It annoys me . . . I just walk out — I don't want to see that woman anymore."

Again he comes back to his bodily cravings: "I just live for eating, drinking, and making love. . . . After a short while, I get bored. This is one of my patterns." Habituation has arrived, and with it comes the inevitable boredom, the emotional body's need for more and more: "I just start with someone else, but I feel a little bit less enthusiastic." The need for pleasure becomes more identified with the sexual need, which also becomes the weapon against boredom, sadness, and neediness — but even that is not enough: "I feel unfulfilled after lovemaking — it leaves a sadness in me. To kill that sadness, I penetrate a woman again; this goes on and on." Even though there was an awareness of the trap he was in, he saw no way to break the pattern, and he died unresolved.

This situation has been repeated in his current lifetime. Olaf has been obsessed with his addiction for sex and the fulfillment of his bodily desires. Where is his spiritual desire? Olaf has recently discovered that spiritual energy in this lifetime and is now using it to help him to clear the addictions to the "quick fix."

The Higher Self brings him important wisdom after his energetic clearing of these themes. It shows him a triangle or pyramid, which symbolizes "the good use of energy." It tells him that "you can use all the sexual energy you want, but it must be used from a point of love, understanding, and enlightenment. It's to be used for your highest good." The message provides him with the missing piece of knowledge that it is not the sexual energy that is "bad" but rather his misuse of it that is wrong — it is the missing spiritual component of love that has prevented him from quickening his vibration to experience "fulfillment" on the transcendental level of spirit.

Once Olaf has explored the first-chakra themes in the Roman lifetime, it is important to go deeper. Where does this sexual addiction originate? Why did he need to experience that lifetime? The Higher Self takes him to China. But this time the point of view is dramatically shifted in order to view sexuality from a woman's perspective. He is now the concubine, who is used for sexual pleasure but does not enjoy it: "I don't like sex, but yet I'm addicted to it." Again the addiction is there: "I have a definite need and craving for sex all of the time."

The first-chakra characteristics — seduction and manipulation, the power struggle of being both the victim and victimizer — are seen clearly in this experience: "When I exhaust him, he often beats me. . . . I just react . . . and suck him dry . . . I'm a manipulator." Eventually she drains him of his energy, and he dies. When the first chakra shuts down, the life force shuts down.

The beginning of this scenario, the rape at ten years of age, is very interesting. Normally one would think that after being raped as a child, sex would be the last thing chosen. But it all makes sense: the sexual trauma is the emotional and physical imprint that demands more of the same. The emotional body is given a potent dosage of stimulant and the addict demands more, so the girl chooses the whorehouse to satisfy the subconscious need. At the same time, however, there are imprints of being victimized by the powerful males — the feelings of helplessness and physical trauma that are associated with the first-chakra memories. So the woman initially seeks protection, but to ensure safety, she must use her power and play the role of seductress (victimizer) in order to survive.

Survival is the fundamental theme of the first chakra. Olaf uses the sexual energy as a means of survival: "[Sex] is my weapon and tool to survive." Competition is also evident: "I must be better in bed than any of his women."

After the master's death she must survive, so once again she calls in her seduction expertise: "I seduce the owner, and he takes me in as his concubine. I do the same thing to him. . . . I seduce him to have food and shelter." Her downfall comes when she refuses the man and is subsequently killed.

This series of events provides an interesting example of the chain of cause and effect. By withdrawing the sexual energy, she then dies because of it. This creates an imprint that will carry into this current life. The emotional body says, "If I don't make the other person sexually happy, I will die." However, the addictive nature of the emotional body also says, "If I don't satisfy my own sexual needs, I will die." Even though this response is not logical to the intellect, it is absolutely real to the emotional body, and therefore the ego holds onto it tightly. The ego doesn't want to let go of this imprint: "It's a matter of survival," says the emotional body.

Another important theme that appears is the need for love. She remembers the brutal rape, and that memory is contrasted with the moments of tenderness and love in the whorehouse and with the master. The need for his attention and the need for safety combine with the fundamental need to be loved, expressed through the sexual act: ". . . if my master doesn't have sex with me, it means he doesn't love me anymore. . . . I need his attention, so to make love is to get his attention." Olaf realizes the emotional-body equation "sex equals love," which is one more theme that is structured into his first-chakra issues.

A key part of this work is seeing who the characters are in this current lifetime. When Olaf was asked by the facilitator at one point who the Chinese master was in the past life, he immediately had a vision of his current wife, Anna. This correlation is significant in understanding the patterns within their marriage now. Whereas Olaf has been consumed with his sexual addiction and, as a result, has had countless affairs, his wife is uncomfortable about and somewhat fearful of sex. It now becomes clearer why this is so. If Anna, being the master, was "sucked dry" and died as a result of Olaf's sexual manipulations, then Anna would hold that memory and would be on guard with Olaf. Again, the emotional body says, "The last time I had a sexual relationship with Olaf, I died because of it!" At the same time, Olaf is needing sex in order to feel love, and because there is little sex with Anna, he continues his search for love elsewhere.

As we can see, a great deal of information is revealed and a tremendous amount of energy is cleared from the emotional body in this ninety-minute session. As the Higher Self brings the experiences to consciousness, the emotional attachments are energetically released. At the same time, the information within the experiences becomes available to help us learn our lessons in this lifetime and put the benefit into action in the world.

As a result of the session, Olaf has experienced a transformation within himself. The sexual addiction has almost disappeared, the affairs have ceased, and now he is finding love in his relationships. The first-chakra themes of power, survival, and control are coming into balance; the clearing of the victim theme, especially through the release of the rape imprint, has opened the energy in his sexual area. The most important change is the flow of the spiritual energy through his body, allowing sex to be finally fulfilling. The search for love has been successful.

As Olaf and others of us clear our deep emotional imprints of the past, the Higher Self will provide opportunities for growth. The sexual energy will be more free to open and rejuvenate itself — the limitations of the past will no longer hold us in old, unproductive patterns. The freedom to discuss sexual issues without judgment and to seek new answers will quickly evolve toward a spiritual-sexual concept of being. The spiritual world will help us resolve the ignorance of the past and create a human wisdom in the future for our relationships. If the sexual energy has the ability to create life, then maybe this energy is naturally within us to empower the subtle bodies as well as the physical body. Maybe there are some secrets about using the energy in different, more powerful ways. It is becoming more and more obvious that we need to break out of the old patterns of sexual practice and infuse more spirituality, more love, more consciousness into our sexual lives. Following are a few ideas that can stimulate the process:

1. Sexual intercourse is about sharing energy in a relationship. The word "sharing" is important because it means the willingness to give and to receive, to communicate intimately on many levels. This energy can manifest on the feeling level as caring, comfort, security, intimacy, playfulness, happiness, trust, sensuality, togetherness, and, of course, love.

2. Sexual intercourse is about opening the physical and etheric channels and letting the sexual ch'i flow, then using that energy to nourish ourselves with its revitalizing qualities. When energy flows, the bodies can more easily come into balance and harmony with each other.

3. Sexual intercourse is multidimensional in its effects and has various purposes for its experience. It can be used for procreation, for sharing emotional intimacy, for physical fun, or for spiritual growth. Consciousness is the key to creating a more profound sexual experience.

4. From a spiritual perspective, we can use the sexual energy to transform the first-chakra need for survival of the species (procreation) to a higher need for "survival": the realization of the Self, which is immortality. To know immortality is to release the fear of death and, therefore, the need for this body to survive. The power of invincibility is thus experienced.

5. Sexual intercourse can be viewed symbolically as a ritual. We can create new rituals to view sex from new perspectives. For example, the sexual act is symbolic of God creating man/woman in his/her image; therefore, the sexual act has the power to create new energy infused with God-consciousness, which can be used for spiritual growth.

6. Sexual intercourse is symbolic of unity, of the merging of the male and female — the yin and yang — energies into a balance.

7. Through the interaction of yin and yang, conception occurs. Conception is the creation of an energy that is greater than the sum of its parts. It implies expansion, transcendence, and the move toward infinity.

8. The experience of "passive orgasm" is symbolic of the silent ecstasy of communion of the yin and yang. This is the moment of transcendence, where two people are fulfilled in a state of nonaction. For the man, this is a state of energy flow

without ejaculation; for the woman, it is also an experience of the flow of energy and fulfillment without an "active" orgasm.

The experience of "active orgasm" is symbolic of the ecstasy that moves the energy toward growing fulfillment in life. Symbolically, orgasm is only a step toward fulfillment. Through the creative act of sexual intercourse comes the energy that, like a seed, holds the potential for holistic development into Oneness. Ecstasy or fulfillment is not the goal of "active orgasm," but rather it is the process, the path of enjoyment, that produces timeless fulfillment in the moment.

Seven

A Case Study of Healing the Victim & Victimizer

I am the twelve-year-old girl,
refugee on a small boat,
who throws herself into the ocean
after being raped by a sea pirate,
and I am the pirate, my heart not
yet capable of seeing and loving.

Please call me by my true names,
so I can hear all my cries
and my laughs at once, so I can
see my joy and pain are one.

THICH NHAT HANH
Being Peace

Maggie was 43 years old when she started her sessions at the Deva Foundation. When she slowly hobbled into the room, it was obvious that this woman had suffered a difficult life: "victim" was written all over her. As the interview proceeded, her long history of physical and emotional problems filled several sheets of paper. She mentioned that coming to us was a last attempt at finding some way to improve her physical condition, because she had spent 22 years working with physicians to no avail. Her symptoms centered around her neck and back, with partial paralysis in her left leg and general weakness throughout her body. For many years Maggie had been practically living in bed, with no will to work and a disgust for playing the role of housewife. Her emotional issues centered on two major areas: her hatred for her father, with its projection to relationships with men, and her dislike of children.

When asked about her relationship with her father, Maggie related a classic story about a strict, alcoholic Alabama state policeman who never had a mother of his own and who chauvinistically laid the law down on how and what a woman should be in his family. His attitude was that a woman was here to obey and serve the man, and he enforced that belief both physically and emotionally. Maggie left home at the age of 20 and married for convenience at 24. She repressed the years of physical and emotional abuse by her father, until finally she was bedridden with the unresolved feelings eating her away from inside.

Her first session exposed an Inner Child full of pain and separation. Since her attitude about children in general was quite negative and judgmental, the Inner Child was full of the insecurity and fear that kept her out of balance. We worked hard at clearing the burdens of emotional pressure, and the Inner Child emerged radiant.

In the second session, the Higher Self took Maggie more deeply into her victim theme, this time exposing her to the perspectives of both roles: here she plays the victimizer as well as the victim. A condensed but literal transcription of that session follows. The material in parentheses represents Maggie's observations of her physical-body sensations as she lies on the table in the session; the bracketed material indicates the observations of the facilitator.

Maggie: I'm a man in the mountains. It is rocky with trees around me. I have on skins like a mountain man and long hair. (My arms are twitching.) I'm perplexed and thinking of what to do. I don't seem to know what to do. [Tears start to come.] I am sad. I have lost somebody who I cared about. My wife died. She was killed in her home down at the foot of the mountain. (I'm feeling strong chest pains.)

Facilitator: *Go into those chest pains and see what memory is there.*

[Maggie now switches roles, becoming the woman.]

Maggie: Now I feel more related to this woman. . . . I'm calm and serene now, but I'm still lying there on the cot in pain, with skins over me. I want to get up, to go outside. It's hard to breathe — I feel a restriction in the chest. (I feel pain going up into the throat and then down into my chest. It's hard to breathe.)

My man is not here — I assume he's in the mountains. He's not here much and I'm lonely. I spend a lot of time in bed. I wish I had some children to keep me company, but I couldn't have any children. They just never came. I'm sad, because of the loneliness. The chest pains come back. They get worse.

He comes home and puts his arm around my shoulder. I feel unhappy because I know I'm going to die. There's sadness and anger because I'm not ready to die yet. It makes me mad. He doesn't seem to care. He knows he can't do anything about it. He's very detached. He goes out and then comes back. He's wondering how long this is going to go on. He's disgusted, not sympathetic.

I feel tension — I'm a little afraid of him. (My neck is getting tight.) [Pause.]

I feel his hands and wrists are tense. My neck gets more tense, along with my shoulders. I try to relax. (I feel my arms and hands are warm and numb, then they start tingling, which increases into a burning rage, like there's a lot of knots in my arms. Now my solar plexus hurts. There's something to do with my hands. My fingers keep moving like they are choking somebody.)

My God, he got mad and is choking me! I'm down on my knees. But I feel like I'm the one who is doing the choking.

[Here, Maggie is in the process of switching roles again.]

I feel anger. [Pause.]

It's over. [Pause.]

I feel relieved, but sad, too. My arms feel heavy, and I want to shake them and get rid of the bad thing that I've done. I'll never be able to get rid of the bad feelings in my arms. [Pause.] I feel guilty now. I know I shouldn't have done that. (It feels so empty.) I can't get rid of this heaviness in my arms. I wish she were back. I kneel down and hold her. I guess I did love her. [Tears.] I wish I could bring her back. I can't. We had an argument, and she made me mad. I try to justify my actions — she shouldn't have done that. I got mad at her for causing the whole thing. What am I going to do now? (There's a feeling of coldness, emptiness, loneliness.) [Pause.]

I try to put it out of my mind. I don't want to think about it. It's the only way I can handle it. . . . Now I'm back on the mountain where all this started.

Facilitator: *Ask your Higher Self if there is anything else to see.*

Maggie: (My neck feels real tight, and my head feels like it has a vise around it. There's pressure on my temples and a tension through my shoulders, neck, and head.)

[At this point, Maggie witnesses her death.]

Maggie: There was a crushing, like a big boulder or rock. I was caught under a big rock, from the shoulders up. I didn't die right away. It was hard lying there not being able to do anything. It was a rock slide. I couldn't get out. It was a relief when I finally died. I welcomed it.

On day three, Maggie came in quite exhausted and full of aches and pain, but there was definitely more light in her eyes, and she was happy with her progress. As she climbed onto the massage table, her physical body led her right into the experience.

Maggie: I feel a pressure in my lower intestines and abdomen, as if something is moving there. It's getting bigger. Maybe it's a baby, but it looks — feels — dark. My stomach is growing. The black thing is still there, like a rock. Now it gets smaller, down to the size of a pea. I don't want it and it goes away. My stomach collapses like a deflated balloon: empty.

Facilitator: *Ask your Higher Self to take you to the source of this experience.*

Maggie: (I feel pain in the solar plexus. My fists are tight, and there's tingling in my right wrist. My shoulders are tight, and there's pressure in my throat.)

Facilitator: *Go into it. What comes?*

Maggie: Father! [It seems as if an electrical impulse is shooting through her body.] I feel fear. I have the impression of a lion. He's standing next to it, and he could care less. . . . [Pause.] Narrow streets and old buildings, like biblical times. He has a uniform with armor on, like a centurion with his lion. I try to maneuver around him, but his position hasn't changed. We haven't taken our eyes off each other. There's a sense of danger. I'm a woman — dark hair, dressed simply. He's guarding the door, so I can't get out. He wears a helmet with an eye guard that comes down. He seems aggressive.

I feel I shrink in stature. I wish I could run through his legs. (I'm feeling a pain in my left shoulder.) I was hit there with his staff. I'm lying on the dirt floor. He hit me. He stands over me, laughing.

Facilitator: *What do you feel?*

Maggie: There's not much emotion. I feel resigned to that treatment. I accept that type of treatment as a usual occurrence. He seems to enjoy doing that. It doesn't bother him to treat me like that. He feels that this is how women should be treated. [Pause.]

I'm sad and resigned, like it is my duty to accept that treatment. That's what I'm supposed to do. I get up, and I'm happy that it's over. I go about my daily business. I'm twenty years old. I don't know where my mother is. . . .

(There's tension in my forearms and hands.) It feels like a rock — hard — like I have a rock in it and I want to hit someone. My left arm seems to be hitting someone, and I'm getting hit back in the stomach and chest. My father is bigger. It's over, and I'm lying on the floor again. There's pain in the chest, like my ribs are broken. He's standing over me, but he's not happy. This time he's really angry, because I fought back. . . .

(I feel intense stabbing pains going all the way through to my spine.) I thought I'd died, but the pain keeps coming back. I wanted to die. He wanted to force himself on me, to have sex, and I fought him off. [Tears, followed by a pause.]

Facilitator: *Take it forward. What happens?*

Maggie: He's standing in the doorway. I'm lying on the bed. I know what he wants, and I can't do anything about it. There's a heat in my hands. I want to scratch, claw, and kick. He's on top of me. I try to push him away, but I can't. He's too heavy. I feel like I'm buried under there — such heaviness. The bed sags. I don't struggle too much any more. I feel resigned. I'll be glad when it's over. I wish somebody would come. I try to remain detached and try not to feel anything. I feel numb from the waist down.

He leaves now, laughing. (My chest hurts to breathe.) I know it will happen again, and I hate that. I hate him, but I feel guilty because I don't think I should hate him, but I do. I feel sick and nauseated. I feel sick with myself for putting up with all of that. I wish it were different. I hang my head in disgust. I wish someone would come in and help change the situation, but I know it won't change. I feel helpless. . . . [Pause.]

(There's a tightness in my stomach. It's growing, like a big basketball.) I'm pregnant, and I don't want to face it. I don't want to see that. It's hideous. I'm blocking everything from the waist down, because I don't want to see it. I'm afraid it will be a monster because of the way it was conceived. I don't want to give birth to a monster like its father. That's what it is. It's getting bigger. It's hideous — a mean black face. It snarls and growls. It fights and kicks to get out. It seems like it is too big to get out. (It hurts to breathe.) I don't want it. It's a thing, not a human, but a black mass. It's alive. . . .

[My Higher Self tells me to have her send the light of the Sun to the entity.]

It's angry. It fights and struggles.

[Maggie goes into a hyperventilating breathing pattern.]

Maggie: It doesn't like the light — it is getting smaller.

[During these few minutes there was a noticeable, almost visible, dark cloud of energy in the room. When the Higher Self began to radiate the sunlight, the cloud dispersed. Within three minutes, the room seemed as if a dozen lights had been turned on, and there was a definite sense of relief.

Maggie: I feel like I've been slit open, like a C-section. There's stuff oozing out, but I won't let it settle down because I feel guilty for losing that baby. I feel guilty for not wanting it. I hate myself for not wanting it. I feel ill and sick at my stomach with disgust over the whole thing. (I've made myself sick because of the way I feel about myself. I wish it were different.)

Facilitator: *Take it forward.*

Maggie: I wish it had been a real baby that I could hold.

(My stomach doesn't feel right.) I didn't get cleaned out right . . . a massive infection . . . it didn't get well. It's deadly. I don't seem to mind dying. I'm too sick to fight it — I feel resigned. . . . [Pause.]

Father didn't come back. I hope he got what was coming to him. He doesn't care what happens to me. [Pause.] I float away.

The following excerpt is from the fourth day of sessions, in which Maggie finally releases her victim theme and begins the process of renewal:

Maggie: My Higher Self comes as a shaft of light. There is such a concentration of light. (My hands are tingling.) I'm way up in the clouds. There's an opening — I see the world below. I see a building in China; it's gold. There's a big Buddha on the right; the building could be a temple. I'm a woman. I see steps going up. I want to go up those steps. It's bright and sunny in there. I sit on this table — it feels cold like marble. (I feel excitement in my body.) I feel happiness, joy. I want to soar — a very joyous feeling. . . . I can hardly contain myself. I want to get out of this body and explode and fly away.

(I feel a tightness in my throat, neck, and head.) I feel the back of my neck held by two fingers. I'm dangling in the air. It may be God lifting me up to the top of the temple. I'm not like a person, but big and white, with a round head, and I'm translucent and getting bigger. If I explode, I'll lose control! My Higher Self creates a big tall tree that I can climb and get out of the top of the temple. I can see all around the countryside. I feel such peace and excitement, like it is too good to be true. I can't believe I'm up here. There's such a calmness. I haven't let go of the tree yet. [Pause.]

I let go. . . . I'm flying — my hands are free. It's bright and soft. I'm lying in the clouds. It feels like I've come a long distance to get here. That's what I've wanted for a long time. I don't seem to be male or female, just a person. [Energy moves through the body.]

Five neon shafts of light are coming out through my forehead — bright blue shafts of light, radiating out of my head and all around it. My whole head feels light, not heavy. My eyes tingle. The light moves down my body. There's a lot of excitement through my body. I'm vibrating. . . . I'm enveloped in the blue light. It's calm and peaceful, like being wrapped in a blue cocoon. There's no pain, no body, total serenity.

At the beginning of each session, we would discuss the details of her previous session so that her mind body could understand the emotional themes that had been exposed and how they related to her present life. Through the understanding of her experiences came additional clarification and an enhanced ability to let go of emotional-body energy. Compassion flows more freely when there is understanding.

In summary, several issues were resolved or substantially cleared during the four sessions. As we have seen, the issues of insecurity, fear, and judgment were so deep-seated that Maggie's physical body reflected them in her paralysis, the shutting down of emotions, and the desire to stay unconscious. The first session opened the emotional body and began the healing process.

Through the balancing of the Inner Child and the opening of the energy flow, her Inner Child/Higher Self qualities became consciously useful.

The second session is interesting because of the symbolic role reversals: starting as the man, switching to the woman's point of view, and then returning to the man's experience. The Higher Self effectively gives a taste of each perspective in order to clear both the victim and victimizer energies as male and as female.

In the role of the woman, there are the obvious themes of loneliness and sadness, but the experience of being weak, physically ill, and in bed most of the time is a reflection of the present-life experience. As a result of her frailty, there is the tension in the relationship and a sense of helplessness in both herself and the man. His frustration accumulates over time until he's forced to seek release or even escape by leaving for the mountains. Her feelings about his detachment and her separation branch into greater tension between them until there is no communication, just repressed feelings.

Another interesting characteristic of her sessions is that the physical-body transformation leads her subjective experience. This means that the body reacts first, for example by her arms twitching, and then the experience emerges in her consciousness. The emotional-body energies detach from the physical body and work their way outward until they arrive on the conscious level of awareness; then the event is seen visually.

The climax comes with the strangulation, which imprints her throat chakra with the judgment of the victimizer — the judgment of male victimizing female, the symbolic act of separation through communication being cut off (via the throat chakra), and her feelings of the helpless victim.

Especially symbolic to the man's role are his hands, which hold the intense frustration and the imprint of guilt. His rage and uncontainable feelings explode out of control and the violent act is committed, which then results in his self-judgment and guilt: "[I'll never be able to] get rid of the bad thing that I've done.

I'll never be able to get rid of the bad feelings in my arms." He makes the promise that he will never again lose control, which means that he will try to bury the feelings and the memories that trigger them: "I try to put it out of my mind. I don't want to think about it. It's the only way I can handle it." This reaction is, of course, Maggie's behavioral pattern today. Symbolically, the big rock that crushes the man is the "rock of guilt" that has trapped her in today's life, that keeps her a prisoner to her unresolved victim/victimizer karmic themes.

After two days of opening the emotional body and moving the spiritual energy through it, Maggie was primed for a major breakthrough. So, as soon as she climbed onto the table, she began to set up the situation for the release. Again, the physical body immediately shows us where the energies are concentrated. She goes into the womb: "Maybe it's a baby, but it looks — feels — dark."

As the body tenses, the judgment energy surfaces: "Father! I feel fear." The most karmic relationship in her present lifetime appears in this past lifetime, with the man again her father and the victimizer, and herself as the younger, weaker female, again the daughter and the victim.

Almost every sentence has symbolic meaning. Not only is this story a classic representation of the struggle between the male and female energies on this planet, but it is also an example of how the body gets imprinted with sexual abuse. How do we usually cope? We either express the emotions and experience the intensity and the pain, or we learn how to repress the feelings, or, more extremely, to turn the emotions off and play dead. Maggie experiences all three. But none of it works, because the emotional body, through the karmic imprints, holds the drug to feed the addictions, and no matter which of these three responses is triggered, it feeds the addictions with its stimuli.

As a result of the rape, she finds herself pregnant. The fetus is the symbolic manifestation of her emotional attachments to her father — the hate, the judgment, the fear of constant abuse.

The feelings are so intense that they create a living reality for her in the form of the negative polarity — the dark, the evil. Her judgment issue is so strong that she has created the embodiment of evil inside herself: "I'm afraid it will be a monster. . . . I don't want to give birth to a monster like its father. . . . It's hideous — a mean black face. It snarls and growls."

The Higher Self is in the process of clearing this emotional energy by first bringing it to consciousness and then symbolically bringing its polarity, the light of the sun, into play. When there is darkness, bring in light. When there is judgment, bring in love. Through the symbol of light and the spiritual healing it stimulates, the energy is transformed.

Multidimensionally, many aspects are being transformed. On one level, the "evil" energy is cleared by the light. On another level, the miscarriage triggers further guilt and eventually death through "infection." The judgment toward her father is so deeply imprinted that it is probably repeated in many lifetimes besides the current one. On still another level, the body holds all these energies and finally lets go. Her mind body immediately recognizes why she has never wanted to have children, because of the unconscious fear of giving birth to a "demon," not to mention her disgust with sex.

After this session, Maggie felt that a thousand kilos of weight had been lifted off her shoulders. The next day, she told me her body was still sore but that she had more strength and sensation in her left leg and in her body as a whole. Within several days, all the paralysis and most of the neck tension had disappeared. Though it sounds miraculous, I feel it makes sense. She had worked hard, and her Higher Self had brought her through hell and back to life. Now she could start living again, which was symbolized in her fourth session.

From the beginning of her session, the Higher Self is obviously present and the emotional body is clearly receiving and radiating the spiritual energy: "My Higher Self comes as a shaft of light . . . such a concentration of light." For the first time her sessions contain a lot of spiritual virtues: "I feel happiness, joy. I want to soar — a very joyous feeling. . . . I can hardly contain myself." She sees herself as a woman in a holy temple, going through an expansion experience for the purpose of breaking boundaries. The Higher Self creates the scenes, and Maggie expands until she can "let go," into the heavens, into the love and light of her true Self: "It feels like I've come a long distance to get here. That's what I've wanted for a long time." As her third eye opens, she is given a vision and a taste of what life can be and will be: "Five neon shafts of light are coming out through my forehead. . . . There's no pain, no body, total serenity."

These sessions are an indication of how much can be accomplished in only four days of work. It is important to realize, however, that Maggie manifested her own healing. My role was to help her understand the process and give her an outside point of view so that she could more easily integrate her pieces of information into the "big picture."

Whereas understanding emotional-body patterns and themes is very important, the most important and beneficial aspect of this work is the energetic releases that occur during the experiences. The mind body may understand, but the emotional body must release its attachments or we still are stuck in the same situation. Maggie knew and even understood why she hated her father, but that wasn't enough to release her from hate. As a result of the emotional releasing, she can now forgive and leave that hate behind her. She's learned many of her lessons quickly through her continuing work on herself, and today she's active and pursuing her spiritual path with great determination and success.

Eight

Our Deepest Karmic Themes

Love is God.
God is love.
Life in God
Is life in love.
To be in love
Is to be in God.

MAHARISHI MAHESH YOGI
Love and God

*A*s we peel the layers of the onion, moving deeper and deeper into more fundamental karmic themes, we will eventually touch the deepest layer. Is there a common beginning point to the karmic wheel? Is the deepest theme common to us all? We must go to the beginning, the Oneness. Whether we view it as our first incarnation or, symbolically, as being born from the mother, our first experience is one of separation.

We come from the light, from the omnipresent unity that many call God. We precipitate into a form from the formlessness; there is consciousness experiencing the birth into the realm of duality, a realm governed by the laws of yin and yang. This "relative" world is a world of change, of movement, of multi-dimensions of energy transiting into matter and back to energy. But the fundamentals of polarity are always seen, no matter how you dissect it. The soul and its expressed bodies bridge these dimensions of creation — the possibilities of incarnated form are numerous. It is doubtful that we begin with a physical body. There is probably time spent in many galactic forms of energy, but it doesn't matter. Even if 99 percent of our consciousness is still unified with the infinite, a part of us is separate. Part of the whole is living within boundaries, and this is the first experience of "life," the first step into the manifest world and, therefore, our first imprint of experience.

On the level of the emotional body, the emotional contrast between unity and duality is at the least irritating, at the most an overwhelming shock. The moment the voice of the emotional body first "speaks," though it be just a thought or a subtle feeling, a thoughtform is created acknowledging the separation from God. Our programming becomes "I'm separate; I'm not God anymore." Somehow we feel different — we see ourselves as separate from everything around us. The beginning of the emotional body's voice of judgment has begun, and with each judgment the sense of separation is increased.

As the emotional body grows and spreads its influence into our other bodily dimensions, our density increases. There is no way to look at this in terms of time, but eventually what we now call the human physical body is created from our past karma.

The energy of judgment always polarizes into opposites. The emotional body attaches a value to this polarity as either "good" or "bad," "right" or "wrong," "black" or "white." Since being unified with God is seen as "good," the feeling of separation then becomes associated with bad feelings and the different variations on this theme: loss, loneliness, disconnection, insecurity, unhappiness, and, possibly, fear.

I recently watched this separation/judgment theme in action.

A client and his wife were having friends over for dinner. This couple had been going through difficult times recently because the husband had admitted to having an affair with a woman named Carol. His wife felt the separation/judgment strongly toward him and was still angry, fearful, and insecure. On this particular night, all was well. Everyone was laughing, having a good time. In the middle of conversation someone innocently mentioned Carol, who was a mutual acquaintance. Instantly, the energy changed so obviously that there was a hush at the dinner table; most of the people, being unaware of the affair, were lost in confusion at the immediate shift from laughter to a feeling of doom. I was amazed at how two people who had been emotionally triggered by one word could instantly transform the feeling in the room. Our hostess, in tears, excused herself from the table and went into her room to cry. The party quickly came to an end.

The separating event becomes the catalyst for many other emotional experiences, all of which can be imprinted within the emotional body, each one an astral thoughtform that can act as a magnet to attract similar energies to us. The emotional body becomes conditioned to "feed" on this energy, like an addict with a drug. For instance, the emotional body stimulates sadness, and the unique vibration of that emotion perpetuates and reinforces that karmic connection within us by attracting situations that result in sadness, a vicious cycle that repeats over and over until a higher energy detaches it from the fibers of the emotional body. That higher energy can come only from the spiritual body, with its quality of orderliness and clarity.

The repetition of separation/judgment experiences causes a narrowing of our point of view, until we are eventually looking through the gun barrel at a world that is polarized into black and white. It is the emotional investment in a personal point of view to the exclusion of other perspectives that is limiting and possibly difficult for relationships. It can block our understanding of other points of view and the feelings behind them. If we are stuck in a self-righteous position on some matter, it will be difficult to empathize and understand what another person is experiencing and trying to communicate to us. For example, if my parents are Ku Klux Klan devotees and have raised me in an environment of racism, where I have been programmed that to be black is to be less human, to be less intelligent, to be a threat, then the repetition of these judgmental attitudes has created powerful barriers to my understanding of black people. This is the antithesis of multidimensional awareness, which promotes understanding of different viewpoints and, therefore, the understanding of different realities.

An effective technique to expand awareness and loosen the grip of our judgments and rigid points of view is what is called the "Reversal Technique." It can be used to look through the other person's eyes to better understand his or her point of view. To start the technique, think of the incident or situation that has triggered your judgment or lack of compassion. Move into the feelings so that the experience is remembered. Then, shift attention into the other person's awareness and experience the point of view *through his or her eyes*. How does it feel to be on the other side of the fence? Can I understand this other perspective a little bit more clearly? What can I learn from this different point of view? Now, open the heart and let the compassion and new understanding flow to release any negative feelings or attachments. This process may quickly and easily shake us loose from our limitations, or we may need to repeat it several times over a period of time until our attached point of view releases, giving rise to an expanded awareness and more pleasant feelings.

It is the nature of the human nervous system to reach out multidimensionally and simultaneously process many levels of information. The spiritual experience of this phenomena is a profound feeling of connectedness, a unity, a *knowing* that expresses more and more of our mental potential. Judgment, however, has a collapsing effect, which forces the awareness into the patterns of karma and into singular perspectives. We must remember that we are here to learn and love, not to separate ourselves into oblivion.

Once we become aware of the separation/judgment theme, we will start to see it everywhere. The world around us, with its history of conflict and war, mirrors to us our own inner conflicts and feelings of separation. Whenever there is conflict, at its basis is a judgment. Wherever there are the emotional-based points of view of "good" or "bad," "right" or "wrong," there is judgment. Even to look at any object of perception and see it as separate, or different, is to be blocked from the ultimate perspective of unity, that knowing that we are all one.

In many religious, spiritual, or New Age groups, there is an addiction to seeing the world made up of different forces of nature fighting each other. We hear about the armies of Satan, the "Dark Forces" led by the "Dark Lords," as well as their opposites, the "White Forces of Light." This is not a teenage science-fiction fantasy, but a common discussion that can be heard today most anywhere in the world. Whether it comes from an age-old religion or some New Age group, it is the expression of the dichotomy within the collective unconsciousness.

Besides being found in the programming of generations of literature, this imprint of judgment is even structured into our everyday language. It is not difficult to think of all the words, all the comments, that subtly perpetuate the theme of judgment daily.

Judgment has been there from the beginning. Will it always exist within us? According to a 1988 Gallup Poll, the United States leads all the countries surveyed in the belief in the existence of the Devil — two out of every three Americans believe in this archetypal evil being. Even former President Reagan called the Soviet Union an "evil empire." The original theories of Karl Marx attempted to dispel hierarchical empires with the belief that equality could be structured within a society where there was no more conflict or domination. Hierarchy implies judgment. But as we've seen, you cannot clear inequality from people without clearing its basis within the emotional body. And you can't clear the emotional body without accessing the spiritual energy.

Dr. Carl Jung spoke of the separation experience also. He believed that the soul of the child — the *Divine Child* — is in unity with God, and that at the moment of birth we begin to experience feelings of separation (from the mother and from God). This sense of separation is continually reinforced within our relationships with parents, friends, teachers, etc. Jung believed that to end the separation, the person must experience a spiritual awakening or feel a connection with a spiritual source. As a result of his work and that of others, many psychologists believe that while psychotherapy can eliminate neurosis or emotional problems, only a connection with some spiritual consciousness will carry the individual into greater levels of fulfillment. This is why the facilitators at the Deva Foundation speak of our work as "psychospiritual."

Judgment comes from the emotional body, but it commonly manifests through the mind body as thoughts of "good" or "bad," "right" or "wrong," and so on. It is important to be able to distinguish between an emotional judgment and the discrimination or discernment of the intellect. We make decisions all day long, but a judgment has an *emotional charge or investment in the situation*. Therefore, we are not talking about a simple disagreement or a difference of opinion (though these thoughts may have a judgment at their basis), but rather an *emotionally triggered reaction* that produces stress in the physical body and constricts the mind body.

The emotional energy of judgment is always self-diminishing and polarized in a stance of separation. For example, in many cultures a tattoo is considered low class or disgusting, a disfigurement to the body. But in many places in Africa, a tattoo is a sign of prestige, a symbol of beauty and honor. The marking is the same, but due to the cultural perspective it is viewed with an almost opposite attitude. Every culture has attitudes and ways of living life that may be different from our own; this diversity is one of the great sources of wonder and enrichment on this planet. When the differences become the basis for conflict, when "different" is seen as "bad" or "undesirable," we perpetuate separation through the energy of judgment. What I wonder is, Why do we want everyone to believe as we do?

There is no way to escape judgment. It is part of living in the world of duality. No matter whether we feel "right" or "wrong" in a particular situation, there will likely be someone who disagrees with us and makes a negative judgment. So the key to living in this situation is to be unattached — to not be overshadowed by another's attitude but to follow our own inner sense of "right action" and move on through life. Personal "right action" may be controversial: One can find people with strong stands on both ends of the spectrum in regard to such issues as divorce, abortion, or eating red meat, for example. Even if in retrospect we can see we have made a "mistake," understanding what that mistake can teach us transforms the mistake into a lesson, so what's the need for judgment? The only need we truly have is to learn the lesson the experience teaches us and the opportunities it provides us.

Any time we investigate the realm of judgment, there surely will be controversy. It's entertaining to watch people give a dozen reasons why judgment is part of life and can never be transcended. They may even say, "But of course there are universal laws. What about the Ten Commandments?"

Chuang Tsu, a Chinese philosopher who supposedly lived in the fourth century B.C.E., also was concerned with the theme of separation/judgment. The following passage from *Inner Chapters* reveals his enlightened perspective:

> Suppose you and I argue. If you win and I lose, are you indeed right and I wrong? And if I win and you lose, am I right and you wrong? Are we both partly right and partly wrong? Are we both all right or both all wrong? If you and I cannot see the truth, other people will find it even harder.

Then whom shall I ask to be the judge? Shall I ask someone who agrees with you? If he already agrees with you, how can he be a fair judge? Shall I ask someone who agrees with both of us? If he already agrees with both of us, how can he be a fair judge? Then if you and I and others cannot decide, shall we wait for still another? Waiting for changing opinions is like waiting for nothing. Seeing everything in relation to the heavenly cosmos and leaving the different viewpoints as they are, we may be able to live out our years.

What do I mean by seeing things in relation to the heavenly cosmos? Consider right and wrong, being and non-being. If right is indeed right, there need be no argument about how it is different from wrong. If being is really being, there need be no argument about how it is different from non-being. Forget time; forget distinction. Enjoy the infinite; rest in it.

Where there is judgmental energy, there is an absence of love. The reason we get uncomfortable when someone talks about the implications of judgment is that we cling to social rules, religious laws, and a concept of right and wrong to give us a sense of security and guidance through the confusion of living. Without a sense of right and wrong, some say, wouldn't we just kill and steal and do all those bad things? If you haven't noticed, people have been doing misdeeds since the beginning of human life. So we created the concept of punishment and guilt — an incredible invention that, in my opinion, has never helped our evolution, except through the letting go of it.

There are three ways to project judgment: (1) from you to me; (2) from me to you; and, the most insidious of all, (3) from me to me, which is self-judgment. It doesn't matter in which direction the energy is directed, the theme of judgment is still the same.

When I judge someone or something, I play a variation on

the victimizer role. I will notice them putting up their defenses in reaction to my subtle or obvious onslaught. Many times a companion theme of judgment, self-righteousness, will be present as well. This attitude says, "I'm right and you're wrong; I'm good and you're bad; I'm the one who *knows* — you are the one who must be taught." Self-righteousness appears when we have become attached to a thought, attitude, or point of view. Because we feel invested in that point of view, we feel we must direct it to others, to "teach them" or "set them straight." We all know that feeling, whether we are giving it out or taking it in. How do we feel afterward? Usually distant, separate, or just plain uncomfortable. That associated feeling can show you that something is not in balance.

When we find ourselves on the receiving end of someone's judgment, usually we feel the victim. There is a sense of threat or of our freedom being impinged upon. There are many re-actions, all common to the victim: fear, anger, withdrawal, sadness. To be judged is to be denied one of the strongest needs a human has: the need to be loved, to be accepted, to be approved of. The frustration incurred by being denied such a basic need can generate a collective reaction like war or programming a religious group to hate another group. Judgment is a powerful trigger point to almost all of the themes in the emotional body.

The most debilitating and destructive response, however, is to *accept* the energy and use it to reinforce our own self-judgment. To judge oneself is *to deny the God within*, to shut down the flow of spiritual nourishment into our lives. The consequence of self-judgment is guilt, and what follows this very sticky and addic-tive energy is the demand for punishment. Here's how it works. Let's say a person has played the role of victimizer and at some point judges himself or herself for it and feels guilt and the need for punishment. Most of the time that person will find a way to be punished, thus reversing the position to one of victim, which may perpetuate itself through lifetimes. I have yet to work with a client who didn't have this system operating strongly — it is part of our cultural ethic. Without belief in judgment and punishment, how would our judicial system function?

Punishment does not dissolve the guilt of the victimizer. I have never seen any healing or release of the victimizer energy by playing the role of the victim. What I have seen, on the contrary, is a person who now holds both. To become the victim does not release the victimizer within — it is a different vibration of attachment. To become free of these themes requires a spiritual answer, not an answer of punishment. Admittedly, it may be an important choice to experience both sides of the polarity, thereby learning a lesson from shifting the perspective. Where, I wonder, did we get this universal theme of the need for punishment, the theme of "suffering for our sins"? Is punishment only a means of personal or social control? How did punishment get into our religious thought? Why do we see God as the judge? These have been personal questions of mine since age six.

Let me tell you a story. There was once a young boy growing up in a conservative home in San Antonio, Texas. On Sundays, his grandparents would take him to the Protestant church, like a conventional family "should." It was a routine that was not at the top of the list of "fun things to do on the weekend" for this boy. On one particular Sunday, there was a guest preacher. He came to warn the congregation of sin, of hell, of anything else that might steal one's soul from the almighty Christian God. The boy couldn't understand all of this talk of sin and evil of the world — he didn't feel like a sinner. This day was really miserable to endure. The boy noticed that he was not the only one withdrawing from the picture painted by this very intense preacher. He closed his eyes, hoping to doze through the rest of the sermon.

Not more than two minutes after he had shut his eyes, however, something started to happen in his consciousness. A feeling of slight disorientation and a flow of heat moved up from his feet. Suddenly everything went white, as if he had been struck by lightning. Time seemed to disappear. As he bolted up in his seat, he became transfixed within a white-light consciousness. There was no church, no thought, no outer awareness — just paralyzing light. He had no idea how long this lasted. Then the light started to flow more comfortably, and he began to relax in its nurturing energy. He heard a soft but clear fatherly voice in his mind saying the words, "God is Love," followed by a pause and then, "God does not judge; only man judges himself."

He slowly awakened to a peace and warmth in his body. It felt safe and good. When he found it subsiding after five minutes, he didn't want it to go away. What did the words mean? His intellect struggled, but his heart understood. . . . I have never forgotten the words, nor their meaning.

Nine

The Healing of Separation/Judgment

When there is division, there is something which is not divided.

TAOIST SAYING

A case study that exemplifies the exposure of the theme of separation/judgment is given by Ann. The following session reveals the multidimensions of what I consider our deepest and the most universal karmic theme.

Ann is an intelligent, middle-aged artist from Fort Worth, Texas. By the time she made contact with the Deva Foundation, she had spent 25 years in psychotherapy, but few of her deep energetic blockages had been removed despite the long process. She was aware of her judgment themes and her guilt, but her main need at this time was to understand the many difficulties she was having with her five-year-old daughter.

Ann: I feel a deep empty space in my solar plexus. It feels like it has been depleted for thousands of years.

111

Facilitator: *Ask your Higher Self to take you to the source of that empty feeling.*

Ann: I'm a nun in a dark brown habit — it's an abusively coarsely woven fabric with nothing under it. It's grimy and horrible, and I tie the belt real tight to mortify the flesh. I never wear shoes. My hair is cut real short — it's chopped off. I'm very thin because I don't eat except some disgusting gruel soup. Whatever is the worst thing to do, I do it. My body is shut down as a woman; there are ulcers on my face. It's so awful.

Facilitator: *Ask your Higher Self to take you back to when you were young to see what happened before.*

Ann: I'm eight years old. I'm an indiscriminate number in a large number of children. I went to the nunnery as a novice because I was very bad: I murdered my little sister. I hit her over the head, but I didn't mean to hurt her — I was just playing mean. She collapsed in the snow. I looked at her, but I didn't know what to do. I was scared to tell anybody — I went and hid. She shouldn't have died so fast — this wasn't supposed to happen. I couldn't believe it — it was so out of proportion to the transgression. Something must be really wrong with me. The Devil's inside of me. I must be a disaster as an incarnate human being and a danger to myself.

I went to my parents and said that I must go somewhere to make up for this. I asked to go to the nuns. They were all like crazy people — they were almost mythical because they were all so far out. They took me in.

[Then Ann moves ahead in time and looks back on the events in the nunnery.]

For a long time I scrubbed the floor. . . . It was always cold — there was no sunshine. By the time I was eighteen, I was into the mortification of the flesh — how far I could go. We did everything imaginable. I'd hit myself with a thorny plant all over my body. These wounds would get infected or develop scabs, and then I'd hit myself more. I would escape from myself as a human. The body just shut down. Then there was sensory deprivation: I just floated in zero, just nothingness. The object was to stay alive — if I died, I knew I'd go to Hell. I was the Devil's possession. Hell is unity with the Devil. It has an intense satisfaction — just as satisfying as Heaven. Everybody thought we were holy, but we weren't.

One day the mountain crumbled all over us, totally crushing the building. A boulder as big as the room fell on top of me. I was crushed. The pain of being crushed was compressed into my chest. I stayed there for a while relishing this. My soul oozed out from the rocks and into the depths, to the center of the earth, to the Devil's caverns. My black badness sank into a molten cavern with the Devil.

The Devil uses up souls like a fuel for his fires. He keeps them for as long as they are of use to him, until they are a shell or a husk. Everything is burned away; then he doesn't want you anymore, and he lets you go.

[Ann now shifts perspective and moves directly into the experience.]

I come out like a steaming geyser: my soul is spewed out onto the surface. It's a forest, a nurturing area. I bring energy into this purified husk and start to incarnate again. It's been a long time of being out of circulation. I regenerate enough to start again. This doesn't seem bad or scary. It's matter of fact to go through this purification process.

My rib cage is tight — it makes me feel sad. I didn't really mean to be bad — it was an accident. It's been a long time for it to finally end. I'm so tired. . . . I lie in the forest. . . . The energy regenerates and rejuvenates my body.

Through this example, the Higher Self shows Ann that the sister who was killed is her daughter today. The Higher Self also gives her the realization that the guilt has carried into this relationship and has associated itself with the feeling of being responsible for the daughter's problems in this lifetime. The pervasive tiredness and emptiness she feels exacerbate the issues.

The irony is that though Ann would push herself to the limits of human endurance, "the objective was to stay alive." "If I died," she says, "I knew I'd go to Hell." As if she wasn't already living in Hell!

It isn't her self-abuse that kills her, but "an act of God" that crushes their building. In the minutes before she dies, she manifests her thoughtform of Hell and the Devil, and experiences what she calls her soul being consumed as fuel for the Devil's fires: "The Devil uses up souls like a fuel . . . until they are a shell or a husk. Everything is burned away; then . . . he let's you go."

Hell is very symbolic, especially the aspect of fire and burning. One interpretation that came up later in Ann's discussion with the facilitator was that it was not the soul that was being consumed, but the karma or "sins" of the emotional body that were being burned as fuel. The conscious Ann was still aware; the "shell" was still existent. The symbolism of the purification is the major theme here, though it is overlaid with the judgment of Hell as the place where evil beings are sent, of Hell as "bad."

The idea that maybe something "good" is happening here finally appears as she is "spewed out" into a nurturing place, like a forest: "I bring energy into this purified husk. . . . I regenerate. . . . This doesn't seem bad or scary. It's matter of fact to go through this purification process." She now chooses the "positive" symbol of a nurturing place, the feeling being that since the "evil" is gone, she can start to be nourished and rejuvenate herself.

Ann's deep-seated emptiness and physical tiredness are symbolically perceived in her solar plexus, the reflex point of the emotional body. She connects with the story toward the end of her life, after years of self-punishment. The feelings are intense;

the addiction to her suffering becomes clearly visible: "Whatever is the worst thing to do, I do it. My body is shut down. . . . It's so awful."

The Higher Self takes her back to see the source of these harsh choices. She sees the death of her little sister due to her mean outburst and her initial disbelief, which then grows into the realization of what she has done. Her self-judgment grows into guilt, which then demands punishment: "Something must be really wrong with me. The Devil's inside of me. I must be a disaster. . . ."

The projection is normal. The ego says, "*I* couldn't have done this. The Devil must have done it — he's to blame." But at the same time, there is the feeling that "I must be bad; if I hadn't treated my sister in a mean way, this would not have happened." Regardless of what exactly was the initial stimulus, the emotional body's themes of judgment and guilt were triggered. That's enough to perpetuate the programming of "I must pay for my sins; I must suffer in order to purify myself of evil. . . ." Of course, once the punishment begins, the emotional body feeds on this new source of energy, and the addiction with suffering begins: "By the time I was eighteen, I was into the mortification of the flesh — how far I could go. We did everything imaginable."

This part is very meaningful, because at the end of the story her choice of nourishment dispels this need to choose suffering. Ann is deciding to incarnate again, to live life, rather than to live Hell. Another irony is that, on reflection, this experience shows the Devil and the little sister as giving Ann a great gift. Without their participation, Ann would not have learned such valuable lessons and had the opportunity to transform herself.

The Higher Self showed Ann that the little sister is her daughter now. By releasing the guilt, she can now release her feelings of "not being a good mother" in this life with her daughter. The tiredness and emptiness can now be filled with energy to live life free of the attachments of the past.

How is it possible to resolve such a formidable karmic theme as separation/judgment? Having been involved in perhaps a thousand Deva sessions where this theme has appeared, I can say that it is wonderful to watch the genius of the Higher Self putting to work basically the same set of solutions time after time.

The first step in the process is to open the flow of energy in the body. Stagnation of energy is no different from the stagnation of water in a river. Just as the eddies and pools of water at the edges of the riverbed fill with discolored water, leaves, and rubbish, so does blocked energy become "polluted." The same principle applies for cholesterol plaque in the arteries and other stagnation-based conditions. Any acupuncturist will tell you that the free flow of energy is the key to health and longevity.

One way to move the energy is with the force of consciousness. Meditation works well over time, but in the Deva sessions, there are various more immediate methods to boost the energy and at the same time open the chakras and parts of the body that have been obstructed. One method includes the use of white-light exercises. The particular exercise that we favor is described in detail in appendix A at the end of this book. Once the energy starts moving, then it is possible to use this flow.

The second step usually is to open the consciousness to the emotional body and start to see what is inside. Once we know what our karmic themes are, it is easier to take action to resolve them. By bringing awareness to their nature and purpose, the healing process is set in motion.

The Higher Self is the best guide to investigate the source, characteristics, purposes, and lessons of our karmic themes. It may take us into the present life to re-experience a memory that has imprinted the emotional body or that has perpetuated an age-old theme. The Higher Self may take us into a past-life experience to reveal the source of the imprint or to start the process of "peeling the onion" to eventually reach the core of a major theme. It may also use a metaphor or allegory to expose the theme — the Higher Self knows exactly what will be perfect for us at any particular moment.

As a result of the Higher Self's healing energy and the expanded consciousness that now sees the purpose, the energetic attachment to the emotional body goes through transformation. A key word here is *understanding*. Through the mind body's participation in the transformation process, we can understand what has happened and possibly why we have chosen it. By shifting the point of view, we change the situation, and two things are accomplished: the releasing of bondage energetically and the growth of wisdom about life. We are never the same afterward. Even the ego starts to trust the process and, more importantly, starts to identify with the Higher Self energy.

So the second step involves accessing the spiritual energy of the Higher Self in order to effectively clear the attachments to the emotional body. Since the solar plexus chakra is the control center of the emotional body, when the spiritual energy initiates the healing process in the solar plexus, the other chakras are stimulated to purify their karmic themes as well.

As the solar plexus opens and triggers the opening of our other chakras, the energy of the body flows with greater ease and power. As a result, the blocked or repressed emotions start to release their attachments and rise into consciousness. At that point, the Higher Self helps us bring understanding and compassion into play so that the emotional themes can be resolved. As this process continues, the third step brings us to the opening of the heart center and the clearing of its themes.

The heart chakra is the center of relationship issues. This includes not only relationships between people but also relationships between the subject and any object of perception. Experience is the energy that links the subject and the object of perception. If a person is not centered in the Self, then an intense experience, whether positive or negative, can be overpowering, which further separates the individual from Self because of the identification the observer has with the object of perception. When this happens, the stressful experience becomes attached to the emotional body, creating a karmic attachment. For example, hearing the news of a close friend's death can possibly create such an overwhelming wave of grief that the person loses a sense of Self and becomes immersed in and identified with the grief to such an extent that it alters his or her emotional life henceforth.

Since the heart chakra holds relationship karma, the heart is usually involved with the imprinting of every chakra in the body, and vice versa: Every chakra is involved to some degree with the heart chakra. We first saw this concept of interrelationship between chakras regarding the solar plexus chakra and its emotional-body control function; now we see a similar function with the heart chakra. These interrelationships likely exist for all of the chakras. Instead of seeing them as independent in form and function, we may be wise to see them as points of interconnectedness and synthesis that act in concert together.

Humanness is an important quality of the heart. It distinguishes human beings from other beings in the universe. To be human is symbolic of "having a heart," and this core theme is probably the one most often chosen to explore by galactic and cosmic beings who desire the human experience. When I say "galactic," I'm speaking of a soul with a deficiency of third-dimensional, "human" experience or a soul that hasn't integrated these "multidimensions of Self" into a human life. The galactic being may be highly developed on the level of mind, body, and the abilities to use energy, but it does not have the unique knowledge of the feelings of love and its expression in relationships. That is why there are so many essentially galactic souls in human bodies now. They are here to learn the gift of the heart.

Being human also includes experiencing the sometimes-painful effects of relationship. Trying to avoid these may be one of the reasons why some people choose to live in cloistered environments such as monasteries, thinking that they can avoid relationship issues there. That's like going to a party and then deciding to lock ourselves in a private room out of fear of what might happen. How much fun is that? For those of us who have come to experience human relationships or those of us who have relationship issues to resolve, it is time to enter the dance and take the risk. We might find it enjoyable, or, better still, we might learn to love, which is the crowning achievement of human life on this planet.

As we look at the relationship function of the heart chakra, our attention is automatically drawn to those people who are important to us: father, mother, siblings, friends, lovers, and those people who are central to this lifetime's toughest karmic lessons. As the solar plexus opens the emotional body to its host of karmic themes, the heart chakra then starts to process and clear these relationships. We start to resolve our anger or heartbreak; we start to understand from other points of view why things have happened the way they have. The heart starts to open again, and the fear of relationship is replaced by trust and understanding. Love starts to flow. At that moment, the evolutionary path has opened to the high road of healing with love. The spiritual frequencies of the Higher Self are now available for expression. The clouds have dissolved in the radiance of the sun.

Once the heart energy begins to flow, it rises into the throat chakra, which immediately begins to melt the frozen themes of judgment and self-righteousness. Where do these themes come from? As I mentioned earlier, I believe their source lies in the beginning, in that first experience of separation from God. As we precipitated into form, that initial experience produced the thoughts "I am no longer infinite; I am no longer in unity!" This was the first judgment, and that thoughtform evolved into the newly created emotional body as the core theme that would always underlie all future karmic attachments. The wheel of karma was created, and we have been moving along that circle for a long time, undergoing every possible experience, learning every lesson life has to teach. Now it is time to come full circle and find the solution for this deepest of our karmic themes: separation/judgment.

The throat chakra is the control center of communication. To communicate is to exchange energy in relationship. It is not restricted to an exchange just between people but includes as well an exchange between a person and the object of his or her attention. We can communicate with anything: a person, a plant, a bird, even a rock. Communication is not limited to a particular form. We are starting to learn and develop its many possibilities. We will discover an ability for telepathic and other psychic forms of communication as we open the throat chakra and clear the blockages to the energy flow.

When judgment is expressed, the first reaction will likely be to throw up a defense to it. No one likes to be judged, and the reactions to it will effectively block any communication, except maybe the communication of conflict. Whenever defensive reactions are elicited, energy is inhibited in its flow, especially in the throat chakra. One explanation is that the basis of a situation of conflict or threat is separation/judgment, and it is that vibration of energy that triggers the closing of the throat chakra.

The most important form of communication is the communication within to the Higher Self. This form of communication can be blocked by the most insidious expression of judgment: self-judgment. This will always close the door to our inner knowing and to the spiritual virtues of the Self. Self-judgment is a judgment on our divine nature, a denial of its reality. If there is great self-judgment, we will have a difficult time relating to the energy of the Higher Self, just as we would have difficulty relating to another person.

What is the answer to separation/judgment? All we have to do is to look at the wisdom of the ages, to listen again to what the masters have taught. We will discover that love is what we are seeking.

In summary, we can say that the heart chakra with its loving energy plays a special role for us at this time in the history of human life. It holds the ultimate answer to all our problems and sets the solution in motion to bring us home to God, to bring us back to unity. Love is that human quality of the heart that always unifies, always nourishes and quickens the vibration, opening the spiritual nature to us. Whereas judgment divides and stimulates the emotional body to play its games, love unifies and gives us the healing solution for the addictions of the emotional body.

People may say, "It sounds so simple, too good to be true." My response is, "What is more simple than our divine nature? What could be more true?" *Love is God and God is love.* When we access love, we are accessing divinity. When we feel love, we are feeling God moving within us. When we love, we are stimulating God within others. We don't "fall in love" — we open our hearts to let the love flow, and the resonance of that universal vibration stimulates all octaves of love simultaneously within others and the environment. Then we choose which octave to express — effortlessly, not from the mind, but from the heart. Since love is God, love is omnipresent, omnipotent. Love has every answer within it, the solution to every problem. To trust in love is to trust God.

As this love energy rises into the throat chakra, its unifying power clears the chakra of judgment and separation. Forgiveness becomes a natural healing expression to the guilt that judgment has created. Forgiving ourselves is another way of saying that we allow ourselves to let go of the deep imprints of self-hate, shame, and other expressions of judgment. As love illuminates the throat chakra, our communication abilities become uninhibited, and we feel the dawning of connectedness. The throat chakra links us to our inner and outer environments, and the love finds multidimensional expression.

As the roadblocks to its flow fall away, the energy continues up into the head, rejuvenating and activating the higher centers of the mind. Most importantly, the love energy, which has now harmonized and balanced all of the chakras, has blended the energy flow into white light. This powerful stream of white light instantly opens the third eye, thereby permanently opening the consciousness to the higher mind. We have reached the realization of the Self, that unbounded awareness of who we are. This wholeness results in the breaking of the karmic wheel. We have transcended attachment: the emotional body has quickened in vibration to such a degree that nothing can hold on any longer.

With the release of our deepest karmic theme of separation from God, we become one again. The ego expression of the emotional body no longer has karma with which to identify, so the ego now identifies with the Higher Self. In essence, it says, "I am the Higher Self!" The important difference between the enlightenment that now has been realized and the moment before the beginning of our journey is that we now can maintain the sense of unity within the diversity. We can be in body, and yet our infinite awareness is permanent. The love feelings and other spiritual virtues dominate our awareness, though we are not without the experience of such emotions as anger or sadness. We have moved to a state where the lower vibratory feelings may still be felt, but without the attachments that overshadow the experience of Self.

In this Oneness, we have become more than the mere collection of experiences — we have evolved. And so God has evolved. All aspects of our being are resonating to make the infinite become more infinite. We stimulate the fabric of creation to expand more and more. We are love, and consciously living that love is the foundation for living.

Hugh Prather, in his book *Notes on Love and Courage*, describes this process beautifully. He says, "Love expands: It not only sees more and enfolds more, it causes its object to bloom."

Ten

From the Darkness Comes the Brightest Light

Man can see his reflection in water only when he bends down close to it; and the heart of man, too, must lean down to the heart of his fellow; then it will see itself within his heart.

HASIDIC SAYING

The good die but live on, in the example they provided.

ADAPTED FROM TALMUD:
BERAKOTH 18B

*M*any people mistakenly think that as we clear the emotional body we release all of the "negative" emotions, and we then live in a world free of hate, anger, fear, and so on. However, these feelings are not like phobias, such as the fear of flying, which once they are released everything is fine and normal and the particular fear is gone forever. What is more true is that it is possible to clear these emotions substantially so that the triggering of those emotional responses becomes less and less; but if we take that to the extreme, then we've become like "Star Trek's" emotionless character, Mr. Spock, or worse, a robot. This is surely not what the evolutionary process of becoming an enlightened human being requires. Our emotions are part of being human, and the expression of them is important to growth.

What about judgment? How is it possible to live a life without being hurt by its omnipresent influence? Can we conceive of a life without judgment? To choose to be born into a human body is to choose to experience duality and, therefore, the separating influence of judgment. The relative world of form is made of the fabric of separation. If it was not, all would be homogeneous, unbounded oneness. To live in time and space is to live and breathe the ever-changing world of diversity and relativity.

The experience of judgment is fundamental to the emotional nature of human beings. We may have released many judgmental behaviors and attitudes, and we may feel a greater sense of connectedness to the world around us, but how close to unity can we take it? We may sometimes feel a sense of defeat because of the seeming omnipresence of the judgment theme or the struggles of even the spiritual masters in dealing with it. If we look at Jesus, for example, we see a man who was a shining example of love and compassion. His life was a great teaching for us about overcoming judgment. But, whereas he may have transcended the judgment of himself and others, there were many who judged *him*. As mentioned previously, the direction judgment flows doesn't matter — it is still the same energy and the same emotional theme. His life demonstrates the profound nature of judgment on the collective consciousness.

This world will always be a world of separation and judgment as long as we incarnate into bodies and choose to work on our karmic themes, but judgment does not need to be an attachment that keeps us separate. It does not need to be a limitation to love and to life. It is possible to live in a world of judgment and not be pulled down into its abyss. We can transform the experience of it and grow from it, use it to open our hearts to love.

A story in this vein that has had a profound effect on me is about a "living angel," whom I shall call Aaron. This man has been a shining example of what I know is possible for all of us in this world.

Aaron was born in a small Jewish village in Hungary in the mid-1920s. All his 63 relatives were devout orthodox Jews, and Aaron started early with his religious studies. He was a yeshiva student, following the traditional religious education of the Jews. As he grew up, he became increasingly serious about his studies of God and the religious law. He didn't have much of a sense of humor, being more focused in his mind than in his heart.

Aaron had chosen a life that would test his faith in the extreme. It began around the age of sixteen when the Germans invaded Eastern Europe and forced the Jews into a ghetto. The conditions in Aaron's ghetto were harsh over the next two years, with little food, unsanitary conditions, and the extreme emotional stress of persecution and death. Aaron watched as some of his relatives died from starvation and disease. It was the first time he had experienced sorrow and loss.

One day he met an attractive young woman, his first girl-friend, and for the first time he felt the opening of love in his heart. They helped each other cope, but Aaron mainly relied on his studies, which he continued with great passion. He didn't understand why this was happening to his people.

Eventually, the roundup came, and his family was marched at gunpoint into cattle cars. After he was separated from his girlfriend, he realized that the rumors were true and that people's morbid fears were actually justified: the unbelievable was happening.

The long-suffering trip to Auschwitz through the subzero temperatures of winter was survived, amazingly, by all of his family. They were fortunate, because many others died along the way. As they pulled into Auschwitz, the collective suffering was like an unspeakable nightmare. The stench of burning flesh filled the air. Aaron tried to stay detached, praying for understanding and salvation, yet always trusting God's will.

As they unloaded onto the selection platform, Aaron held his two-year-old brother in his arms and walked in front of his father. Aaron didn't know what was happening, but his father noticed that anyone holding a small child was immediately sent in one direction, which consisted mainly of the old and weak. All of the strong men were sent in the other direction. As they approached the selection table where the infamous Nazi Mengele sat, Aaron's father said, "Aaron, give me the child quickly!" "No, Abba [father]," Aaron replied, "I'll carry the baby." His father demanded quietly, "Do as I say. Give me the child now!" and he took the baby out of Aaron's arms. As they stepped up to the table, Aaron and his older brother were sent to the left, while his father, his baby brother, and his weak mother were sent to the right.

The next day Aaron asked where his family was being kept and discovered the truth: that all the people sent to the right had been taken to the gas chambers. At that moment, he realized that his father had knowingly saved his life. His father had understood that the Germans would not risk panic by trying to separate a child from a family member's arms, so even a strong boy who was holding a baby would be sent to the gas chambers in that situation. Aaron experienced a surge of energy through his heart as he felt his father's love for him, which was so strong he would sacrifice himself to give his son another chance at life. His father's love was stronger than his need for survival.

At this time, most people would have projected out their pain in the form of hate and judgment. Aaron did not. He found solace inside himself and in his steadfast faith and trust in God. His religious belief that God gives each of us a time for life and a time for death helped him handle the death of his family members and others.

Aaron was assigned to one of many factories to work as a slave. The work was almost constant, and they were given little or no food to provide strength. Yet in spite of all this, he was amazed at the great acts of love that he witnessed all around him. One person would share his or her own meager portion of food with another; someone else would give a gift of clothing to one in need; another would share a blanket for warmth. There were constant words of love and encouragement to provide some support through the long days of struggle.

One day Aaron noticed a single blade of grass. It was the first green plant life he had seen in more than a year. Because of the starvation, anything green was usually immediately eaten: grass, leaves — all vegetation within the camp and the surrounding area. But Aaron carried this single blade of grass around with him. It became an object of love, his connection with nature. Through the blade of grass, he could connect with a world of harmony and balance. In a moment of celebration he shared the blade of grass with his older brother, and they ate it together.

Another event had a profound effect on Aaron as well. After being confined to his barracks one night, he found his bladder painfully full. Since he wasn't allowed to leave for the latrine, he urinated into a tin can and then threw the urine out the window. Unbelievably, he heard a scream of rage and realized that he had thrown it on a German guard! Fully knowing what would happen next, he prepared himself for a quick death. The soldier threw the door open, his rifle extended, and screamed to know who had thrown the urine out the window. Before Aaron could open his mouth, a man who was lying next to him, close to death, said he had done it; instantly he was shot.

Aaron was dumbfounded: Right in front of his eyes he had witnessed yet another act of great love. It seemed that in the midst of all this suffering and abuse, every day he saw acts of kindness and lessons of love that were beyond his immediate comprehension. His mind didn't understand all of it, but his heart was starting to fathom the world of God and love in a time of hell on earth. His belief system had structured a reality that was producing miraculous changes within him. His reality was being continuously infused with reminders that even when the darkness is extreme, there are those who share their light of godliness with each other; that even through hate and condemnation it is still possible to love and give everything, even one's life, to help another person. Aaron began to believe that it was his destiny to survive and share his love with others. As a result of so many incidents of extraordinary giving, his heart had become fully open.

He wondered if it was possible to love the guards. He made the attempt, but it was too difficult — he couldn't do it. He did, however, realize that whereas he couldn't feel love for them, he could have compassion for their position and eventual fate. He felt no hatred, and whatever judgment existed had changed in quality. He judged the *acts*, but he no longer judged the person committing them. His compassion and understanding had grown to such an extent that it melted the attachments of his emotional body. He realized that these were ordinary people who, under extraordinary circumstances, were performing inhuman acts. The addictions of their emotional bodies (judgment, hate, being the victim or victimizer, etc.) were playing out scenarios that have been seen countless times throughout history.

As Aaron's heart opened, he continued to create opportunities to express his love and caring. He felt a deep connection to his fellow prisoners and slave laborers. He would tell them Hasidic stories and try to comfort them with his humor and spiritual inspiration. Their suffering was great, and his compassion was great also. He was now "in relationship" and expressed his love openly, which could be dangerous, but his Higher Self, that eternal "witness" to life, reminded him of the spiritual lessons he had learned and comforted him with the feeling that God would protect him. As time passed, he somehow continued to survive the growing number of roll calls where thousands were sent to their deaths.

One day Aaron heard a rumor that 500 people would be sent out to Auschwitz to a coal mine in Germany. He was excited at the chance of leaving this place and having another chance for life. The roll call came, and as they lined up, Aaron's brother held Aaron in front of him in a protective embrace. (His brother was so tall Aaron always felt cared for.) His brother said, "Aaron, you stay in front of me so I can see you. I'll watch over you." When the count was made, Aaron was number 500. His brother and the others were sent to the gas chambers. Again and again Aaron witnessed his destiny, which seemed to be survival, and the great acts of love that were given to him as blessings.

Aaron was forced to work hard in the mines, but fortunately one day the Germans left the area and abandoned the prisoners. The Allied Forces had arrived, and Aaron was free. He was alive, but weak and with nowhere to go. Life was still a struggle, but now he could start anew. He still witnessed the persecution: no one wanted these starved and haunted Jews. People were concerned only for their own survival in a land devastated by war.

He had one distant hope in his heart. Before his family had been taken to Auschwitz from his village, his older sister, Rachel, had been separated and taken away by the Nazis. Aaron wondered if she had survived, so he wandered through the countryside searching for her. As he walked through an American sector, he asked two Americans if they could give him a ride in their jeep to Hungary. They agreed, but said they had to wait for a translator to join them before they could leave. Aaron was sitting quietly in the jeep waiting for his ride when suddenly out of the door walked his sister, who was the translator! It was an incredible moment. After so much that had happened, he felt God's love complete within him. Sixty-one relatives had died in the Holocaust, and he was now reunited with the only living member of his family. His only hope had been fulfilled.

Aaron and his sister immigrated first to Israel and later to America, where they live today. He still gets up before dawn to practice his traditional prayers to God. and he continues to thank God for his life and to thank those many people for their gifts of love.

This is a story of one man's path to love and God. He could have chosen hate and judgment: He could have blamed God for the destruction of his family and his people. He could have felt abandoned and chosen death, but instead he chose life and the love of God. He surrendered to God's will and never let go of his trust. Within the suffering and the darkness, he discovered his greatest treasures. Today he still radiates that knowing that nothing can touch him, that God is within him and around him. That security will never be taken from him. He owns it and emanates it to all he meets. He is an example to all of us of the power of love to transcend judgment.

The following Hasidic prayer encapsulates the elements of Aaron's — and our own — drama:

> *A person may come to sense two kinds of movement*
> *taking place within him as he prays.*
> *At times he feels the left hand of God*
> *pushing him away;*
> *at other times God's right hand draws him near.*
> *But even as he is pushed away,*
> *he should still know*
> *that this is only for the sake of his return.*
> *Even as he feels*
> *the might of God's left hand upon him,*
> *he should see*
> *that it is God Himself who touches him.*
> *This too he should accept in love,*
> *and trembling, kiss the hand that pushes him,*
> *for in that very moment,*
> *the right hand awaits his coming near.*

My wife, Paula, has always been a marvel to watch as she processes her emotional-body issues. One of her deepest issues has centered around man's inhumanity to man, exemplified by the Holocaust. Her judgment themes have woven into a complex web of guilt, pain, sorrow, and fear. She has faced these issues repeatedly in her past-life work and "peeled the onion" to the core. But it was her specific confrontation with her pain over brutality issues that was truly remarkable.

As a child, Paula had an intense fascination with the Jewish culture and often dreamed of the Middle East, of deserts, and of biblical times. As soon as she was able to read, she began to consume any books that she could get her hands on that dealt with the Jews. She was raised Episcopalian and later taught Bible study in a church, but it wasn't until her twenties that she felt the freedom to convert to Judaism. She chose an orthodox conversion, which initiated a full immersion into living the life of a Jew. She took on one Jewish project after another, engaging in a full range of work from teaching to politics.

The project that dominated her attention for approximately eight years was the education of society about the philosophical, theological, socioeconomical, and political causes and consequences of the Holocaust. She traveled through Israel, the Soviet Union, and Eastern and Western Europe *except for Germany*, doing research for a documentary film on the Holocaust. She wrote, produced, and directed a film for use in high schools, universities, and churches, and she used it in her many lectures to the public. During this time, she also served on the board of directors of an international Holocaust organization with Nobel laureate Elie Wiesel.

Though she was certainly processing her karmic themes, the pain she felt deep inside was not alleviated. She could not bear to be with Germans on German soil — her judgment and fear were evident. Germany still represented the "unspeakable" to her, and the fear of "Nazi consciousness" continued to hold her in its grip.

Later, after Paula started to commit herself to a new direction in her life and made a decision to return to therapeutic work with individuals, she began to open that locked door of deep judgment issues. In an incredible past life, she first saw herself as a two-year-old child who died in Auschwitz.

Before the time of her death, she spent many cold and hungry months in a Polish ghetto, until she and her parents were shipped in cattle cars to the death camp of Auschwitz. Her last memory was of being held by her mother as she was walking down the train platform toward the men who were leading the selection process. When asked what happened next, her Higher Self responded that she died in her mother's arms in the gas chamber. As a result of this revelation, coupled with years of study and teaching about the themes of the Holocaust, her emotional body released another layer of the victim/victimizer theme, and due to the law of resonance, the karmic connections to all her other unresolved issues started to transform themselves. As we say, "her stuff came up."

Shortly after this breakthrough, I planned our first trip to Europe to work with a long list of eager clients in the Munich and Frankfurt areas. Paula never said a word about my decision, and, of course, it never occurred to me that this would be a problem.

Two days before we were to leave, Paula came into the room crying and said that she could not go to Germany — it was too much for her to handle. Her past memories gave her feelings of anger, fear, and judgment. It was obvious that she was in pain and that we did have a major problem, so we discussed the situation at length and meditated on it. After several fluctuations between "Let's go" and "I can't do it," I finally succeeded in getting us on the plane. It was difficult for me to watch her go through the constant challenges of her emotional body. And it didn't get any easier once we had landed in Munich. Paula kept feeling "Nazi energy" all around her. I could almost hear her thoughts: "I wonder where that man was in 1943?" "I wonder if this man was a Nazi?" Anyone over the age of 60 was suspect. Even driving on the Autobahn was difficult — Paula would see a sign for Nuremberg and Dachau, and it would trigger memories, anguish, despair, and tears.

Fortunately, we were staying in the home of a young woman

healer. She invited us to a healing meditation given by several German healers. During the meditation, Paula broke down into tears as she let all her pent-up emotions out. She felt a sudden sense of compassion, understanding, and love surrounding her. The anger, fear, and judgment that had been alive in her for so long was melting away. She explained what was happening to her, and the people responded with even more love. It was so beautiful — I couldn't even talk because the tears had choked me up.

I think all ten of us were in tears. Paula thanked everyone and told them that after experiencing their closeness to God and their dedication to the healing life she could now let go of her fear and her judgment. She communicated that her issues with Germany were just a projection of her fear of her larger karmic issues. She could now be free of them. Paula had manifested these truly loving, kind, and gentle beings to help her resolve her theme of judgment.

Two days later, we attended a healing ritual at the concentration camp in Dachau, which is just outside of Munich. I was worried that this might trigger another wave of judgment and pain for Paula. We were met by four other healers from Germany and Europe. I watched Paula carefully and noticed how full of light she was. Love and forgiveness radiated from her like sunlight. She was emotional, but this time it was the emotion of healing and growth. It was an inspiration to watch. She gave her traditional Hebrew prayers for the dead, and we could feel the energy lifting, the power flowing through her — it was obvious she would never be the same. This trip to Dachau had been a test by her Higher Self to see if she could put into action those changes that had taken place within her emotional body. She passed the test with flying colors!

I somehow knew that from that moment on, she was complete with one of her deepest themes for this lifetime. It was a great lesson for me because I had watched the process over the sixteen years that I had known her. This evolutionary force has been confirmed repeatedly by watching my clients heal the impossible.

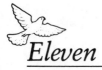

Eleven

Gurus, Channeling & ETs

*There is but one guru
and that is God.*

BHAKTI SUTRAS OF NARADA
(pp. 25–30, 45)

What are the fundamental qualities of being human? Some say that *desire* is at the core of our lives and that the inability to fulfill desire creates frustration, pain, and desperation. Desire is born of the spiritual need to be in God, to be one again. The feeling of separation pushes us to want the most: infinity. Therefore, separation is experienced to motivate us to search for ways to be in unity with God — to feel the communion, to know that perfection. As a result, we have demanded someone to play the role — a Jesus, a Krishna, and so on; someone to tell us what is right, to show us the way; someone to have faith in because of our personal deficiencies. Because of the core separation/judgment theme, we never feel perfect; we don't feel worthy of the gods, though we create hierarchies to attempt to move closer to God. The question arises, Is it really possible to reach a state of enlightenment?

It is undeniable that most people are suffering in a state of nonfulfillment. This suffering is due to the conflict between our need to see ourselves as good and loving and our judgment about ourselves that we are never good enough. Approval from others is important, as is the feeling of being worthy, of acceptance of Self in the moment, yet our judgments keep us from enjoying that approval even when we actually allow ourselves to receive it.

According to the Bible, "God said, 'Let us make man in our image, after our likeness.' . . . So God created man in his *own* image" (Gen. 1:26–27). One interpretation says that this implies the connection and unity of man with God. Man was chosen to mirror God's image, to be a reflection that was perfect. The human form was created with the thoughtform of man in unity with God. However, the church dogma has emphasized the idea that man has "fallen" and, as a result, is born in sin. This programming may be another way of describing the separation theme: that man has fallen out of unity with God. The mind body may understand the connection with God, but the emotional body identifies with the separation imprint.

We have long been raised with the idea that to be enlightened or even to be highly spiritual is to be *less human*. Jesus is represented as the only son of God, who is more God than man. Then there are the Krishnas and the pantheon of deities of different cultures around the world, who again are on a "higher" level than man. Personally, I find the stories, the mythologies, inspiring — up to a point. When we see being spiritual as coming into conflict with being in a human body or having human emotions, then we have introduced a detrimental judgment theme of "I'm not good enough" or "I can't help the fact, but I'm *just human*" or "To be human is to be a sinner."

In many religious orders, the "human" aspect is shut down, turned off, controlled, denied, flagellated, and so forth. Some people believe that if we destroy the humanness long enough, we will finally transcend into purity. This is one of the obvious themes in Ann's past life. The truth of the matter is that we either "descend" into *unconsciousness* because we can't handle the torture any longer or we exit permanently!

For most of us, however, it is the subtle programming of human as *separate* from God that affects us in our daily lives. The constant judgments, impatience, lack of compassion, and so on are just outward signs of the problems within. The criticism of ourselves and others only reinforces the experience of separation within us and does not solve the problem. But the acknowledgement of our humanness as a blessing *will* move us closer to God. In fact, it is said that the angels are jealous of our human opportunity, because humans can evolve so quickly by being in these dense physical bodies and having the experience of emotions. We have the machinery of perception that can experience life and the environment to grow into oneness in this lifetime.

There is so much to be thankful for in human life. We are blessed with such richness of thought and feeling, from the depths of total despair to the heights of ecstatic unity; from the simple intelligence of a newborn baby to the realization of "I am"; from the calm peacefulness of floating in an aquamarine ocean to the power and thrill of the expansion of consciousness. We have it all — the opportunities for growth are virtually unlimited. Yet we often do not realize that there is a perfection in all things. The painful feelings and experiences are just as right for us in the overall pattern of our lives as the experiences of love and happiness. Our choices are perfect because they indicate what is needed for our evolution at any particular moment.

Related to embracing our humanness is the need some people have for a guru. There are many types of teachers, but the spiritual teacher is supposed to be enlightened, the perfect example of knowledge in action. There are a few enlightened teachers in the world today, and it is wonderful to feel their presence and to listen to their wisdom. These true gurus are not just teachers but the living example of liberation: a reflection of the unified trinity of God, Guru, and Self.

There are also masters who are not fully enlightened but who have mastered one or more dimensions of knowledge. This is the norm, I have found. The purpose of such teachers is to pass on the teaching, to be the open channel for all "students" to learn what they individually need for their own growth. When teachers use their status to control others, this constitutes a misuse of power and a betrayal of purpose. Guru means "teacher," not "tyrant." The teacher who does the job effectively connects the student with the master teacher within. This process disengages people from the attachment of giving away their power to the enlightened guru.

The teaching of surrender is many times misunderstood to mean "defeat" or "giving our power away." To learn surrender is to learn to let go of our attachments and limited perspectives. This process brings us to a place of freedom and open communication with the Higher Self. Therefore, the true guru helps us release attachment — even to the guru.

This tendency to give away our power — our trust in our own truth — is a common problem today. It is found not only in the ashram or in association with many gurus today, but in the corporate world also. The traditional "military model" instills the belief that the boss knows best, that he or she has "the answer." The emotional theme of judgment reinforces that belief, saying, "I don't know enough; I'm not smart enough; therefore I'm not good enough," thus creating a situation that breeds dependency and irresponsibility, and perpetuates the helpless victim theme. Fortunately, the old corporate model is beginning to crumble as new leadership roles are being explored. The new model is saying that the true leader's role is to *empower* others, not to *control* them. Spiritual values are beginning to penetrate this traditionally "bottom-line" world.

We must recognize that while the acquisition of information and experience from others is important, the development of consciousness and the knowledge of Self is essential for the evolution of any human endeavor. To have knowledge of Self is to be in harmony with natural law; therefore, creativity is without hindrance, and the power can be utilized without fear or chance of abuse.

At the Deva Foundation, the facilitators are often asked, "What do you think about Carl Jung, Edgar Cayce, Joseph Campbell . . .?" There is a human tendency to confirm our opinions with someone who we *perceive* has some "better" knowing or more "advanced" understanding than we ourselves do. We often forget that every person has at least some unique kind of brilliance and genius of expression. We may see their wisdom in their smile or the sensitivity of their insight. When their perceptions and point of view interface with ours, we can share their knowledge free of confusion and noise. It is at that moment we are blessed with a gift of confirmation of our own knowing. There is no need to judge how wise or enlightened they may be; all we need to do is to open ourselves to the acceptance of the gifts that are offered, those gifts that resonate, that touch us deeply. We need to realize that the energy that doesn't connect with us is meant for others or exists merely for the benefit of the giver, which is also very important.

There are a lot of people waiting for the Messiah, waiting for an incarnation of God (as if we don't have God inside of us!) to come rescue us, to take us to heaven, to confirm our faith that there is salvation. Personally, I hope that the Messiah never comes!

For a divine being to come rescue the planet would mean that the thousands of years of growth and learning would be a failure. Mankind would not have learned the most fundamental lesson: that we *are* God! We can do the job ourselves. This is the final chapter to ages of struggle — we are learning the final lesson. We are realizing our divinity, and we will, *collectively*, transform suffering into liberation. That's why if you meet the Messiah on the road, tell him he's not needed here, ask him to please let us revel in our dawning accomplishments. The Messiah is within our own consciousness — the Christ is not a person but an awareness of divinity. Now is the time for its glorious manifestation from each of us. But, before that can happen, there is work to be done: The attachments of the emotional body must be released. Once that is accomplished, we open the channel to love, the great healer, and love is God.

Another variation on the guru theme is seen today in the widespread popularity of the channeling of disincarnate beings. Because of the flashiness of such experiences and because this phenomenon is quite surprising to people who are just entering into the world of spiritual possibilities, channeling is seen as acquiring truth from the "guru in the sky." Many times the information that comes through is prediction-oriented, saying that this planet is due for a major catastrophe — natural or man-made — which has sent many scurrying to "protected" areas here and there. My question is, "What does this have to do with spiritual growth?" Fear may be a well-tested technique for the dictators of the world, but not for supposedly spiritual leaders, whether in body or not.

What concerns me the most is *the need of the emotional body to hold onto dependency and powerlessness*. We have a Higher Self inside with all the answers and with the perfect formula for success. Let us channel our *own* knowing — we don't need another entity's opinion, unless it is part of the plan of the Higher Self and the energy is taken through the filter of the Higher Self's knowing. This is like using the Higher Self as an energy transformer to adjust the difference in frequency between you and the entity.

Where did we get the idea that just because a disincarnate being is "on the other side" it is omniscient? If it does have some valuable information to give us, how do we know that the human channel is clear and we are getting an accurate communication? One point to remember is that no matter how evolved an entity may be, that entity is not ourselves; it is not our Higher Selves. Only the Higher Self knows our karmic choices and the path we each are following. An entity can make mistakes. Hundreds of clients have come complaining that they were told this and that and it didn't happen. Hopefully, the real purpose of their experience was to learn the lesson that we should look inside ourselves for the answers we are seeking.

Some of the entities channeling to large groups have interesting reputations. The fans are proud that their entity is five thousand years old and lived on Earth at a time when life was different. Other proponents boast that their entity comes from the Pleiades or Andromeda and that it has never been in a human body. My response to them is, "Then why do you think these entities know anything about being human and living on Earth now?" I see unhealthy symptoms of spiritual codependency in these relationships. What I say is, "Entities may come and go, but the Higher Self is here forever." (This would be a great lyric for a country-western song.)

At the Deva Foundation, we are having some fun with the current interest in channeling. We have created a new service, one that will specifically benefit other members of our families who have been neglected for far too long. I'm referring to the millions of house pets that also have karma and are pursuing a spiritual path to dog and cat heaven on Earth.

One of our Deva Foundation facilitators has been blessed with a cat named Idaho, who channels not one, but several, enlightened cat beings: Felix the Cat, Morris the Cat, the Cat in the Hat, and Fritz the Cat. To the best of our knowledge, no other animal has been blessed with this gift. Even though this is undoubtedly a rare opportunity, the Deva Foundation, with great appreciation, is charging only $25.00 for a one-hour channeling. For this small fee, Idaho the Cat will channel for your pets that pertinent information they need to be happier and more enlightened companions. It is important to understand, however, that this tape-recorded session will be understood only by animals. This is not for humans, because you will not hear any words on the tape, only the psychic vibration that will liberate your pet. But don't worry, the peace and harmony that you will experience from your pet will spread through the entire house and benefit everyone.

(We have just received a late-breaking flash regarding Idaho the Cat. She has broken through another psychic barrier and is now also channeling *Lassie*! So tell all the dogs that were uncomfortable with cat entities that Lassie wants to talk to them, at no extra charge!)

On a more serious note, another phenomenon that seems to be occurring much more frequently these days is extraterrestrial (ET) encounters. I have noticed a higher percentage of clients who are being "contacted," not to mention an increase in media attention. Interestingly, many of these encounters are not the stereotypical UFO experiences, but, instead, they are unique communication contacts on the level of consciousness. People are reporting experiences that occur during meditation or sleep, or of awakening in the middle of the night to a contact that may be either "flashy" or more subtle. All the recipients would swear by what has happened; many have noticed significant changes in their lives afterward.

For example, I hear reports that the "close encounter" experience may produce a radical shift in consciousness. One client says, "I always felt that if there would be some contact with an ET, it would be incomprehensible and full of confusion and communication problems. But my experience dissolved that misconception. I had the distinct feeling of connectedness, a fluid flow of understanding that gave me a new sense of universality. Life now is less threatening, more synchronistic and psychic. I have a greater trust in the universe, as if I'm supported in a way I've never experienced before. It's like someone is watching me."

Another person describes her experience as "immediately creating a feeling of expansion and unity with all life. The heart opens and the love I feel connects me with everything." New Age teacher Ram Dass describes it perfectly by saying, "When the heart is open, one can hear the whole universe." Regardless of the experience, most of the encounters I have heard discussed produce tangible changes that are integrated into the consciousness of the person.

My own personal experiences, plus what I have been told has occurred with some forty to fifty clients, lead me to believe that the ETs are not flying in on their psychedelic saucers but are interfacing with us from other dimensions. Like all beings, we are multidimensional, and now we are learning how to be "awake," to be conscious of many dimensions at once. Our only limitations emotionally have been due to our programming, which judges and says extraterrestrial contacts are insane — "good, decent people don't talk and hold hands with galactic light forms."

The fact that these ET encounters are happening more frequently implies that we are clearing the blockages that have arisen from our limited points of view and have kept us from accepting these experiences as real and meaningful. This creates the possibility for multidimensional communication with the ETs. As the throat chakra continues to clear its themes of separation and judgment, these experiences will become more normal and widespread. We will move into a conscious multidimensional life, gathering and processing information and knowledge on many levels simultaneously.

Of course, we could get attached to extraterrestrial information as easily as we can get attached to channeled-entity information or to any information that comes from outside ourselves — the situation is basically the same. Generally, we see the entity as being the teacher and the human being as the student.

I suspect, however, that in many of the recent ET experiences the roles have been reversed. If these ETs are bridging dimensions in a search for more understanding, which is evolution in action, then maybe we are experiencing "reverse channeling." They may be choosing to contact people who have an extraordinary knowledge and wisdom; or even more likely, given that the ETs usually fall into the "galactic" category, which implies great development of the mind but not of the heart, they may select a person who has a developed heart chakra, a person of great emotional sensitivity and love energy. This fully feeling human would be a perfect being for galactics to connect with in order for them to understand the workings of the human heart, which may be needed for their own evolution. Even without the person's conscious knowledge, there may be a mutual agreement between the human's Higher Self and the galactic beings that permits the access of human experience and knowledge.

I am convinced that this process happened to Paula over a two-month period. Almost every night, extraterrestrial beings would come and learn from her — it was just another Deva Foundation class, though admittedly unusual! This interaction with extraterrestrials is one more reason we are fortunate to be on Earth now. Let us welcome all beings here — we have so much to share with and learn from each other.

Just as fascinating to me as these unusual ET experiences are the inner experiences of what I will refer to as "good ol' boys." For one thing, it is somewhat rare to have the opportunity to put one of these conservative, conventional, beer-drinking Republicans on the table and look into the emotional body for current- or past-life imprints — normally they would steer a far course away from such a "questionable" practice! But I must say that what has come out of such sessions has been pleasantly surprising.

One of the most interesting past-life sessions I have heard about is that of my father. Probably partly out of curiosity about "what in the world his son is doing for a living" and partly because of encouragement by family members, he decided to come and do four sessions with Paula. It is important to understand that my father doesn't have an esoteric bone in his body. I heard a friend ask him if he had ever heard of Edgar Cayce, and my father responded, "Yeah, didn't he play for the New York Yankees?"

Let me give some background here. As a result of growing up in San Antonio, Texas, and living there all of his life, my father knows a lot about oil, hunting, and sports. He essentially made his living selling insurance and playing gin rummy at the local country club. So, as you might imagine, he is a Texas good ol' boy who wouldn't know a chakra if it was spinning right in front of him! I must applaud him for having the courage to get on the table and do the sessions. What was even better was that he had no trouble with the process — Paula could barely write fast enough to keep up with him! The following is an account of his fourth session:

Paula: *Ask your Higher Self to take you into a lifetime where you experienced spiritual energy, power, or purpose.*

Wendell: I see a lot of sparkling white buildings, white stone streets. Everything is made out of this white stone, like marble — it's pearlized or like white shell in appearance. There doesn't appear to be any wood or timber in this architecture, but there is a lot of glass. The sky is luminous. What the hell is this place? I have no idea where this is — I've certainly never seen anything like this before!

Paula: *So let the scene unfold and speak out what's happening.*

Wendell: There are big cracks in these buildings — they are everywhere. There are people, but they seem unconcerned about these cracks. What the hell is going on here?

Paula: *What do these people look like?*

Wendell: An interesting thing about the people is their uniformity in physical and emotional characteristics. There aren't any real short or tall people, there are no deformities or ugliness, and everyone is so graceful in their movement. They never rush or panic. This is a really weird place — this isn't anything like Greece or Rome, even though everybody wears robes or togalike clothing. These people seem so content. I can't understand why there are cracks everywhere! [Pause.]
    All the buildings have a similar architectural configuration. They are different sizes, but the building on the hill — it feels like a temple — is the biggest: a square with a circle in it, a dome within the four walls. It seems the higher you

go up, the bigger the homes, but the same general shape. The temple holds a great power within it. I can't define the power, but it feels like a deity. . . . That energy radiates through the community — the people feel taken care of by it. . . . Maybe that's why everybody seems so happy with the status quo. [Pause.]

Paula: *Ask your Higher Self what role you played in this community.*

Wendell: There seems to be a distinction between classes. I'm part of the teacher/priest group. There seems to be a dress code — the highest class of people are dressed in the purest white. Other classes wear a light blue, a light yellow, a light rose; you know, there isn't any green or brown around here. . . . What is this place? Where am I getting all these pictures?

Paula: *What else is happening?*

Wendell: These teacher/priest people seem to float or levitate when they move around. This is really weird. I teach, I explain about the subconscious, about imagination, about science, etcetera. I am hairless, and I'm wearing a snow-white toga or gown. There is no evidence of cold weather or extreme heat — it's like everything is under control. Our food is fruit, vegetables, fish. . . . I don't remember any animal life with the exception of those strange regal cats with yellow eyes. They're not aggressive, but very watchful with those penetrating eyes. [Pause.]

Paula: *Take it forward to see what happens.*

Wendell: The end came when there were earthquakes, serious tremors. Now I understand where all those damn cracks came from. . . .

The city, our land is surrounded by water — there is no land in sight. This is the final destruction: it's falling into the sea. The streets lead down to the docks. There are three boats waiting there for the people. They're shimmering in the sun with golden light. . . . I calmly lead the people down to the boats . . . like a guide. The quakes are getting more severe. The different classes of people are all evacuated to the ships, but not us — the white-robed class. We remain to face our end in the sinking city. My task was to lead the people to the ships.

My father is an example of how each of us holds a greater richness of experience within than superficially meets the eye. Whether or not what he saw is an accurate description of a real past life, Wendell tapped into the universal collective unconscious and brought forth many points of connection with the Atlantis myth. The fascinating thing is that before the session my father had no knowledge of Atlantis. As he said later, "I never used the word Atlantis in my recall. Any association between Atlantis and my story is your assumption. But those cracks sure were real!"

This is not the first time I have seen people go into lifetimes in previous historical time periods and describe them as if they were historians discussing their research. The Higher Self can give anyone access to those memories that are important to us now, in this world. My father admits that this "Atlantis" memory has unlocked many doors to his inner world and has shifted his "conventional" point of view tremendously. For the rest of us, it shows that even good ol' boys from Texas may have a few surprises up their sleeves. We should not be too quick to judge by outer appearances!

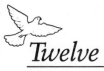

Twelve

Love
& Unity —
Synonyms

May all beings exist
*   in happiness and peace.*
Great compassion makes
*   a peaceful heart.*
A peaceful heart makes
*   a peaceful person.*
A peaceful person makes
*   a peaceful family.*
A peaceful family makes
*   a peaceful community.*
A peaceful community makes
*   a peaceful nation.*
A peaceful nation makes
*   a peaceful world.*

BUDDHIST PRAYER

*A*s I sit down to write this final
chapter, I become immersed in another beautiful morning on the
north shore of Kauai, Hawaii. The ocean has an incredible way

of expressing every shade of aquamarine as it reaches out to join the horizon of blue meeting blue. Yet to hold the water in the hand is to see its clarity of no color; the same is true for the air around us, but the reality doesn't diminish the beauty of our perspective.

In Kauai, one is aware of two colors, the blue of the water and sky and the green of Mother Nature — their intensity is quite powerful. This island is called the "Garden Isle," and it looks like one would imagine paradise to be. As in New Mexico, the devas of nature are expressed almost tangibly here; there is less of a gap between the subtle and superficial levels of nature. It's why people come here to rejuvenate and release their tensions. Nature takes care of them as they take care of themselves.

I awoke early this morning with a feeling that something special was going to happen. Paula and I arrived here yesterday from Molokai, another island of special energies. Our house sits on the beach near the Na Pali wilderness area, at "the end of the road." The only sound is that of the waves greeting the land. The only people are those in an occasional boat passing to see the magnificent cliffs and waterfalls throughout the Na Pali coast. Occasionally, you can see the dolphins jumping and spinning through the air as they play joyfully with each other. It's a perfect place to maintain the connection between inner and outer divinity.

As I meditated this morning, the silence and peace created an immovable foundation within me in which to structure thought from the deepest levels of consciousness. Pure and simple, each bubble of thought manifested on that platform of mind. I felt like I could just sit back and witness energy being created and then transmuting into matter, to a tangible thoughtform. I felt the Higher Self within me and around me, but at the same time holding my hand. At times I would see its face smiling with that quality of friendship and love that always makes me warm inside.

Then the thoughts that had been coming singularly and symbolically began to flow — thoughts of God, of the need for God in a world of struggle and strife, and about how we can move quickly into an age of enlightenment.

I have always felt that the solutions to the world's problems must begin with the smallest unit of society, the individual. Our governmental and social programs can improve the current conditions, but for lasting change to occur there must be a renaissance within each person. The obstructions to global enlightenment must be removed by the input of a powerful dose of spiritual energy. Only a higher energy can shake us loose from our sense of stuckness. I believe that this spiritual energy has to come from the reservoir of light and love within each of us, not from outside ourselves.

I adhere to the "hundredth monkey" theory: that it takes only a small percentage of "light bearers" to kindle the light within others. As more people radiate orderliness, the disorderliness is neutralized. As we reach that phase transition point within society, the movement of life on Earth toward the realization of God will be exponential — there will be an immediate shift into an enlightened world. The dream will manifest. The sun of truth will no longer be obscured by cloudiness, and all will see it and feel it warmly.

In the meantime, our planet is crying out in pain. Our "outer body," the environment of planet Earth, is being degraded and polluted at such a rate that it is not unlike a body that has been traumatized and is going into shock. Because of our personal pain and disintegration of body, the planetary body is experiencing the same abuse. Our life force of primal elements — earth, fire, water, and air — is being quickly destroyed! The ch'i of the earth is sick, and it will take time to stop the degeneration and then to rejuvenate. If we don't begin the healing process soon, it may be too late. It is time to acknowledge our inner and outer suffering, to feel the broken heart. From this experience can be born true devotion and the motivation to work hard for healing. As the Jews would say, "Let us never forget." Let us truly learn the lesson!

The technological abuse of power by the masculine energy has been the major contributor to this condition: the victimizer must let go of the karma of harm. The feminine energy of the earth must now rise and release the gauntlet of the victim theme, letting its nourishment and love heal our wounds. When the masculine energy sheds this abuse-of-power syndrome, which has been raging out of control throughout the universe for aeons of time, then that power can be transmuted into the invincible energies of love and compassion, that magical balance of the yin and yang energies.

This process begins with the individual. As we each deal with our own victim/victimizer themes, we can transform those thoughtforms that are still alive and well within our emotional bodies. These themes will not just disappear — expansion of consciousness is mandated. Our Higher Self knows how to resolve these age-old imprints; we must now ask within and listen. The answers are there, and the work must begin immediately.

As we work on ourselves, it is necessary and very appropriate to work externally on our "outer body" as well. The society and the environment can be treated symptomatically while our core imbalances are dissolved on the level of consciousness.

Every teacher or healer will agree that through the sharing of knowledge or love, the giver receives as much or more than the recipient. As Tom Wilson, in his lyrical way, says, "Love is the only thing you get more of by giving it away."

It is from my work with clients that I have learned most and achieved my greatest healings. As more people share their resources with others, the resources themselves will grow, creating more and more consciousness and love. It is time to extend a helping hand and to treat ourselves, others, and our planet with loving kindness. We are not separate: We are all part of the Oneness. This is the ultimate perspective.

So many of our problems arise from limited perspectives, from those attachments that constrict our point of view and bind our sense of the boundless. Let us instead expand — no matter in what way. Let us imagine an awareness that could encompass billions of light years of space. Let us study astronomical scales to shake us loose from the small and constricted. Let the consciousness stretch, fly through the hundreds of billions of stars in each galaxy, and then move through the countless galaxies.

Could there exist beings that are so advanced, so highly evolved that their awareness could span such an infinity? The incredible answer to that possibility is that *we*, Homo sapiens, have that potential and, furthermore, we have come to do it *now*.

A transformation occurs to our limited perspectives upon witnessing a death experience or a miracle like levitation or the healing of a "terminal illness"; something happens to the astronaut who looks from the moon to beautiful Earth moving effortlessly through its cycles, or to the person who has a direct experience of God or one of the infinite mysteries. What is it in the experience that changes us? Could it be the touching of the deepest fabric of being, bridging the conscious mind to that taste of Self, that catalyzes the shift?

The opening of an infinite energy into our previously closed system of body-mind and the consequent quickening of the frequency of our etheric cellular life force initiates a natural process that is always waiting to be activated. After the experience of opening to higher energy and the resulting expansion of consciousness, we then etherically and physiologically stabilize and integrate that higher octave of energy flow. As a result, the brain coherence becomes then the new platform of "seeing," "realizing," and "actualizing" the ultimate perspective of God-awareness. This is truly an experience of the numinous, that nonrational but profound sense of holiness, an awe that transcends the initial separation into a unity experience. It is time to seek this experience and claim it, because it is our birthright!

One of the most powerful transformations I have observed in our Deva sessions is the unity experience. This is literally one of the many God-realization experiences that occurs when our consciousness opens into unboundedness and expresses the innate knowing of God-consciousness. The highest vibrations of the spiritual body penetrate into every level of our multidimensional nature, which produces a unification of being. For this state of consciousness to become permanent, the emotional body must release all of its attachments to karma. Then the Higher Self gives us our diploma of graduation with the bliss of enlightenment.

Even before graduation, it is possible and very beneficial to experience the feeling of unity and live a taste of utopia. The Higher Self can shift our consciousness into that coherent state of vibration and hold it there until the outward stroke of purification rushes forth. As was mentioned before, when the emotional body starts to vibrate, or spin, at a higher rate, then the heaviness of our attachment to the karmic themes separates and falls away. However, this "unstressing" process can be full of uncomfortable emotion or physical release — rarely when we are vomiting the poison do we simultaneously feel bliss!

Many times the Higher Self chooses to manifest a God-experience in order to break loose a deep karmic theme. The idea that "the greater the intensity of the light, the deeper the descent into the darkness" has been confirmed innumerable times. The inverse is also true: The deeper into the darkness we penetrate, the more light we manifest.

The second is the more common experience seen in sessions. The Higher Self wastes no time or opportunity in plunging into the emotional issues in order to clear the darkness. I particularly admire these clients who work so deeply, because this takes courage. But everyone on the planet will move quickly into the situation where unity becomes real and no longer a dream of what life can be. When people are given the taste, they will no longer be bothered by doubt; their feet will be firmly set on the path, and they will have the push they need to accelerate down the path of evolution.

One example of a unity experience took place in a session with Celeste, a German woman who came to the Deva Foundation with the goal of clearing her feeling of isolation in the world and her fear of male domination. She had played the role of victim all her life, continually putting herself in situations that perpetuated the theme, especially regarding strong-willed men.

After four sessions on four consecutive days, she had cleared many of her victim/victimizer issues. She worked hard, with great determination, and received the benefit of greater understanding and peace within herself. I noticed that her body was no longer bent over and tight, that she could stand straight with an air of dignity and strength; but most apparent was her ability to finally look people in the eye with love and compassion. The fear was gone. I gave her two days to contemplate her four sessions, and then we met for a final session before she was to fly back to Germany. This session was completely different from the others — it was what we call a unity session.

Even before I was ready to sit down and start the session, Celeste began her experience, which follows:

Celeste: My Higher Self has appeared as Shiva in masculine form, dancing, swirling, full of light and energy spinning off from him. It is so powerful, yet it feels heavenly light, not heavy or overly intense. My body seems to spin with him — I feel my body becoming that light . . . my hands and feet are tingling with electricity. For a moment I feel a bit concerned about all this power, but now I know it is great. [She goes into silence for two to three minutes.]

Now Shiva seems to be in a feminine form with many arms, all holding flowers. She's smiling a smile that penetrates into my heart. . . . I feel my body fill with warmth. [Her physical body stops vibrating. She becomes calmer.]

Now the Shiva form seems to merge both the male and female aspects into one, and a new form is created . . . like a youthful, androgynous Krishna figure. He or she is so beautifully radiant, as if Krishna is the incarnation of pure love. There's not a judgmental bone in the body . . . just love, so much love. [She goes into silence for two to three minutes.]

Facilitator: *What's happening? Speak it out.*

Celeste: This love is dissolving me into it. Krishna holds my face and I feel a million volts of electric love flow into me, but it doesn't overwhelm me — it just fills me up. [Pause.] Krishna takes me into memories of this present lifetime. . . . [For ten to fifteen minutes she reviews her memories.]

I feel that I can see the true meaning of all these memories. It's true — I feel like I can see from another point of view . . . there's no more judgment about all of this. I look at my father and instead of hating him, it's as if I can see his Higher Self; he's full of love also. I see myself with him, but it is as if I'm in him and he's in me. My Higher Self says that we are one, that he's made of the same spirit that I am. When I look at his face I see my face, a reflection — it seems so real! My mind can't handle all this, but my heart understands, my heart knows. . . . This is great!

[Pause.] You know, everything really is one. . . . I see myself everywhere, in everything.

Krishna is in view again. He comes to me. I see my face reflected in his. I don't even feel he's different . . . we are one. This is what it's really about. I can't believe this . . . this is so incredible. God and man are one, all is one. Now I understand what my Higher Self has been teaching. It's so simple. [Pause.]

I feel myself expanding. I put my arms around the Earth and give it a big hug of love. You know, if we would just give each other a hug like this . . . our bodies would learn how to merge . . . to feel the unity.

My Higher Self, Krishna, has now changed form again — it's me, it's really me! I feel the merging with that Divine Form. . . . I know I will never forget this! I just want to be in this.

Facilitator: *So just be with it; let the body remember it.*

Celeste: I feel real good. [She rests for thirty minutes.]

The rarity of the unity experience in our life and around us in the world does not mean that it is not there for the claiming. Our programming and the tyrant of the ego have kept us blinded for so long that we have come to believe that darkness is the reality and that light and love are the dream. If we have been raised in darkness, with the window shutters closed to the light outside, then we can only stumble around in the prison of that darkness. We can choose to light a candle, which, though it is not the sun, is enough to teach us about life and give us some freedom from being overwhelmed by the darkness. Once our point of view has shifted, we can begin to use the light to find a way out of the room. We open the shutters, and the brilliance of light irradiates us, but even then it will take some time to adjust to the intensity of the light before we jump out the window.

In this transition time, let us start to see the many manifestations of light, learn how to use them, create more, and shed our attachments to the darkness. Let us also thank the darkness for its teachings, which allow the light to give us an understanding of polarity and its purposes. Let us look for nature's examples of balance, of the inherent unity within the diversity of creation. Let us learn another thousand ways to show our love; let us be awake and receptive to what our relationships can teach us about merging, trust, oneness — about how to create a love, a God, that is permanent in our awareness and that radiates a demonstration to our world.

To set our intention is to set our direction homeward to Self. To break apart constriction, we must give of ourselves, and that will start the energy moving again. To choose fulfillment is to choose to be in the present moment — it is the only moment that is real. The Divine Child knows how to live in the moment, to be simple, and how to live in unity, free of judgment and separation. Now is the time — on all dimensions — to realize that emerging Divine Child and come home to Self.

I close with a prayer that helps me on the journey:

A Prayer to My Higher Self

I speak to my Self, in my Self, to know my Self.
I allow my true Self to guide me. . . .
Allow me to unfold like the flower
So all Nature can share the smell of sweetness.
Allow me to radiate the Light like the Sun,
To bring Light into the darkness.
Allow me to understand that all Light flows from a
*   common source.*
Allow me to let the Light shine from my heart into the
*   heart of others.*
Allow Nature to offer me the gift of balance and
*   harmony,*
So I can live in unity in this world of diversity.
Allow me to be aware of my judgments and take loving
*   action to release them.*
Allow me to give understanding when there is doubt,
To extend trust when there is confusion,
To see the lessons when crisis occurs.
Allow my path of life to be the path of love and
*   compassion.*
Allow me to be here now.

As I write these words, I manifest a symbol to enrich my faith. A white dove lands on the back of a chair in front of me. I sit in astonishment, just looking into its eyes as I feel a thrill vibrate through my body. . . .

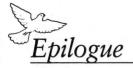

Epilogue

*I*t is a time to bring heaven to earth and let people know that fulfillment is possible *now*. Therefore, we chose for our foundation the name Deva, which means *divine* in Sanskrit. A deva is synonymous with an angel, but more specifically, it is a nature spirit that represents a manifestation of the fundamental laws of nature. We have chosen this name because it represents returning to the naturalness of all things.

We have located the Deva Foundation in a secluded valley high in the Glorieta Pass in the Sangre de Cristo Mountains near Santa Fe, New Mexico, and we have built it with the spiritual force of love. This beautiful area lies in the middle of a sacred spiritual sanctuary that is alive with the healing spirit of nature. The healing devas are almost tangible, as if they are calling each person to take one more step toward divinity and experience heaven on Earth.

The sessions we offer are designed around the specific needs of each individual, and they provide unique and immediate approaches to clearing the limitations to life in order to experience freedom. This holistic system does not ignore the physical or mind bodies, but rather it balances and integrates our multidimensional nature through the energy and guidance of our inner knowing, the Higher Self.

Being a charitable organization, the Deva Foundation is dedicated to manifesting resources in order to put them to work to raise the consciousness of the planet by directly and financially supporting those people and projects that serve our world's highest interests.

We have heard the saying "Give a man a fish and he eats

for one day. Teach a man to fish and he eats for a lifetime." The Foundation is putting this wisdom into action. One such project is helping to finance the education of a Thai woman who is studying organic farming in Japan so that she can return to Thailand and teach her people what she has learned in order to better feed themselves.

In addition, the Foundation is providing educational programs, seminars, workshops, and publishing to share our knowledge and experience not only with those interested people of the world but with those healers and practitioners in search of expansion. We have completed two three-month, in-residence training programs as of 1989 to teach our work to those people who are interested in new and innovative techniques for psychospiritual development. Besides fulfilling the need in society for this type of clearing work, the trainees move through their own personal transformational experience during their time here in New Mexico, which provides them enhanced experience to draw from while working with clients. After graduation, they return to their homes as Deva facilitators and offer sessions in their own areas. We have facilitators in Europe and Scandinavia, as well as throughout the United States.

Appendix A

A White-Light Exercise

White-light exercises are used for the purpose of moving energy through the body with the power of consciousness. The following exercise has worked well for our clients, and therefore I recommend it. It is not necessary to do it for long periods of time —even five to ten minutes is enough to energize the body and clarify the awareness.

This exercise can be practiced either sitting up or lying down with the eyes closed. After taking a few minutes to rest and be with what is happening inside yourself, allow yourself to breathe deeply for three to five minutes, then start the exercise:

1. Bring a stream of pure white light from the universe into the heart, and let it expand with this spiritual energy. Let the heart become full, so that it overflows with love and light.

2. Allow that love and light to flow up into the throat, nourishing and opening the throat chakra.

3. Take the light up into the head, filling it with this light of clarity; allow it to stimulate the higher centers of the mind and radiate a stream of light out of the third eye. . . . Feel it open; feel the expansion. Be with that for a minute. Then draw the light out of the top of the head, opening the crown chakra. Radiate the white light out the crown chakra and fill the room with light. Be with that white radiance for a minute.

4. Now come back to the heart chakra and draw in more healing light; then draw that light up to the shoulders, down the arms, and out the hands, radiating it out into

the room. Feel the flow of love and healing, and radiate it to the world for a minute.

5. Come back to the heart and draw more white light in, and circulate it through the rest of the body. If you notice any blockage or tension, concentrate the healing light on that blockage and feel it clear.

6. Once the body is glowing with light, allow the light to flow to the solar plexus chakra. Push it through the emotional body and out the solar plexus, radiating the light into the room. Feel the light open the emotional body. Let the love and light flow from the universe into the body, and then radiate it back to the universe. Be with that feeling for a few minutes.

7. Take a minute to be in silence before opening the eyes and getting up.

I feel that it is important at this time to emphasize the heart chakra. The chapter on judgment (chapter 8) explains my theory in detail; this exercise is an extension of that theory. By taking the love and light from the heart chakra up into the throat and head, we begin a beautiful balancing process. The heart directs our deepest yin energy into the head (which contains predominantly yang energy). This yin energy will help activate our psychic abilities and deep spiritual consciousness.

As we take the light to our shoulders, down through the arms, and out the hands, we are guiding the energy along the existing heart and pericardium "Envelope of the Heart" acupuncture meridians. This will stimulate the flow of heart ch'i through the body. We are assisting the efficient flow of "life blood" from the heart to the body.

The last step of pushing love and light through the emotional body is representative of opening the chakra of the emotional body and radiating energy out, instead of sucking it in. The complete process is a perfect preparation for contacting our Higher Self or "just being in the flow."

White light is our divine nature. We are not separate from it, though we may not be conscious of it. This exercise helps us to become more conscious.

Enjoy. . . .

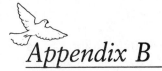

Appendix B

The Transformation Session

> *Does the caterpillar dream of becoming the butterfly*
> *and flying freely? Or is he content to wander the*
> *leaves, satisfying himself on their nourishment?*
> *Maybe the caterpillar must first transcend*
> *within the silence of its cocoon to bring its dream*
> *to consciousness and then to manifestation.*
>
> RICK PHILLIPS
> *December 1987*

One of the special meditations I have developed for my clients is called the "Transformation Session." It is based on a universal nature symbol, the transformation process of the caterpillar into the butterfly. I have found that the application of these fundamental laws of nature in the symbolic form of a guided meditation can connect and align the subconscious with the harmony of nature. The use of all of these steps of transformation can remind us of how easy and natural it is to change, and that change is part of life. The wisdom of the butterfly is there for us to use, to help us when life becomes stuck or rigid. This meditation can aid us in moving the energy again, to put us back in the flow of life, allowing Mother Nature to guide us.

There are five major steps to the Transformation Session:

1. Preparation with white light;
2. Nourishment of the caterpillar and creation of the cocoon of transformation;
3. Transcendence to the silence of Self;
4. Transformation and the liberation of the butterfly;
5. Living in freedom and final unity with the Source.

There are several ways this Transformation Session can be used. It can be done alone by learning the steps and then practicing them. It will take a few times to effortlessly flow with it, so another possibility is to record the instructions on a tape, and then use the tape to guide you. You also can have someone facilitate the process for you. This can be fun and powerful, because both people will be contributing energy and sharing the experience.

The session can be done as often as you feel comfortable doing so. It is most effective when you need a little push to make a change in your life or when you feel stuck. It can be done at the beginning of each season to allow you to naturally flow with the changing seasonal energy. Or it can be done just to connect with Mother Nature, which always feels wonderful.

If you have any questions, you can write to me at the Deva Foundation. Also, there are Transformation Session tapes available for $10.00 apiece, which will lead you through the experience naturally and effortlessly.

Transformation Session

Draw a stream of white light from the base of the spine up through the vertebrae, at first going slowly so that you can feel it move through each one. Take the light all the way up to the neck and into the back of the head; then let it come out from the crown chakra until it is right at the top of the head. As it streams out of the crown, let it radiate out a foot or two, and then bend it like a figure eight and bring it into the third eye. Feel this twist of the energy, and then plunge it right into the third eye. Then pull the light into the middle of the brain and let it flow down over the front part of the body, moving first over the throat chakra to open it, then down to the heart, opening it. Keep moving the light, down through the solar plexus, opening the emotional body, and then down through the sexual area to the base of the spine. Then bring it back up the vertebrae as you did before, letting it radiate out the top of the head, into the third eye, down the front to the spine, then up the vertebrae again as you continue the cycle. After you do this once or twice slowly, then do it more quickly. Breathe in as you bring the light up the back, and breathe out as you take it down the front. Take a couple of minutes to practice this part of the exercise.

Next, move the energy outside along the sides of the body. Starting at the left foot, bring it up the left side of the body to the head, around your head, and down the right side so that it circles, or spirals, around the outside of the body. Let that continue for a few minutes.

Now, as the energy spins around you, visualize a funnel of light going into the heart. Allow yourself to spin with it, moving in smaller and smaller concentric circles until you go deep within the heart to that point of silence of the Inner Self — that place of silence where you can just rest. This is like being at the bottom of the ocean, where the water is very calm and quiet. Be with that stillness for a few moments. . . .

From that source of silence within you, allow yourself to create an energy that manifests a beautiful forest. See the forest full of tall green trees, very lush, very beautiful. Notice the different shades of green as the sun filters through the forest. Allow yourself to experience the energy of the color green.

Allow yourself to focus on one leaf of one tree; see the green, and allow yourself to come into form as a caterpillar on that leaf. As the caterpillar, allow yourself to take the nourishment of that leaf into your body. Green is the color of balance and harmony; it is the color of nature. Allow that green to expand you, to allow you to grow, to develop, to mature. Go into the growth process and take in that green nourishment. . . . Feel what's happening.

Feel your body — does it feel full? Now that you have taken the energy in, go deep within yourself and create a thread of light; draw that thread outward. Start to spin it around your body; feel the silken threads of light spinning from your feet up to your head so that you can create the cocoon of transformation. Experience the light as very delicate, very beautiful, infinite and strong, spinning around and around your body.

Go into the experience of being inside the cocoon — feel the safety, the protection of this energy, the security inside. There is no fear, just the feeling of being easy and simple and effortless, so that you can draw inside yourself, so that you can leave the material body behind. Go inward to your source. Allow yourself to go inward into that silence of the Self, into the infinite, to that which has no boundaries, that which just *is*. Meditate for about ten minutes inside of that silence. . . .

Now, in that silence, bring into you that light and creation, that energy for transformation. Pull it into your physical body. Allow the light to fill you up, to begin the transformation — to create that person you want to be, to create your image as a reflection of your spiritual nature, that Higher Self energy. Feel the cocoon full of light. Feel the caterpillar begin to transform into a butterfly. Feel your body change; let the Higher Self energy transform you.

When you are full of light, allow the cocoon to break open. See the light rushing out as you emerge from the cocoon. Spread your wings and fly like the butterfly. Feel yourself lift off; you are no longer limited to the earth — you now have the freedom of the heavens. Feel the freedom of flight. Feel how much fun it is. Take a minute to experience this state. . . .

Follow your instinct as a butterfly, and fly to a big field of wildflowers. See what flower attracts your attention. What color is it? Land lightly on that flower, and move inside the opening and connect with the energy of that flower. Draw the nectar of that _____ (any color) flower into your body; taste its sweetness, feel its nourishment. Feel the strength that _____ (color) gives you. When you are full, then fly to another flower; see what color you choose now. Repeat the experience with the second color. Keep flying to differently colored flowers until you have covered every color of the rainbow; take every color, every vibration, into your body until you are full and complete.

Realize that you are not just taking in *their* energy, but because of the perfect balance of nature, you will give the gift of creation to every flower you touch through the pollination and fertilization process. So, as you are receiving the nectar, you are also giving the touch of creation to the flower; and through the process of reproduction you thus help create more flowers, for all the butterflies and all of nature to enjoy.

Now allow yourself to fly high, full of energy. Look to the light and fly toward the Sun. As you fly closer and closer, feel the warm and loving energy of the Sun, the giver of life. As you approach the Sun, feel all of the boundaries fall away, feel the natural expansion . . . into fullness. You are coming home to your source, to your true Self. Merge with the Sun; feel the unity, the oneness. Be with that experience for a minute. . . .

Now, full of light, feel yourself radiating that love and light of the Sun, giving that energy to the universe. Also give that light and love to Earth.

Realize the connection between the Sun and your tree in that green forest. The Sun is the creator of life on Earth, the source that provides the green energy on the leaf that the caterpillar drew inside his body, which gave nourishment . . . which was used to create the cocoon of nourishment . . . which allowed the butterfly to be born and to break free and fly into life . . . so the butterfly could share energy with the flowers and the whole world . . . and then fly home to the Sun: the perfect cycle.

Allow your body to remember this cycle, to imprint the knowing of this process of transformation — to know how to change effortlessly and grow toward infinity.

Rest in the Sun now. Be the Sun and radiate that energy always. . . .

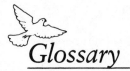
Glossary

ACOA: Adult Children of Alcoholics.

AKASHIC RECORDS: The linear, chronological record of memory imprints, including our incarnational history.

AROUSAL LEVEL: That state of excitation of the nervous system. A high arousal level is characterized by excitement and hyperactivity; a low arousal level is characterized by tiredness, boredom, and hypoactivity. The optimum condition is when the nervous system is in a balanced state of arousal.

ASTRAL BODY: A nonphysical subtle body that contains the lower emotional body and, therefore, the karmic imprints and memories.

AURA: The electromagnetic field generated by our chakras, which emanates from the etheric body.

AYURVEDIC MEDICINE: The traditional medicine of India. *Ayur* means life; *Ayurveda* means the science of life.

CHAKRAS: The electromagnetic energy centers of the etheric body that spin at different vibratory rates, which produce the colors and integrity of the aura.

CHANNELING: The flow of information or consciousness from our Higher Self or, commonly, from another nonphysical source through the vehicle of a physical body. An example would be the trance channeling of spirit guides.

171

CH'I: The ancient Chinese term for a nutritive subtle energy that circulates through the acupuncture meridians.

CODEPENDENCY: An addiction or emotional attachment to a person or a relationship and the problems this brings. This set of learned behaviors may develop into a situation of self-diminishment and neglect.

COLLECTIVE UNCONSCIOUS: That set of subconscious memories, karmic themes, and universal truths that belong to humankind in general.

DEVA: Means "divine" in Sanskrit. Commonly synonymous with angel, especially as a nature spirit.

DIVINE CHILD: An aspect of the Higher Self that carries the spiritual energy of the initial childlike state into manifestation in the physical body of the child or adult.

EGO: The voice of the emotional-body attachments.

EMOTIONAL BODY: An aspect of the astral body that is the container of karmic imprints. Its lower-vibration voice is called the ego. The higher emotional body is an aspect of the spiritual body, as it expresses the so-called spiritual virtues of joy, bliss, love, and so forth.

ETHERIC BODY: A nonphysical subtle body that links the physical body to the other subtle bodies and contains the ch'i energy of the acupuncture and nadi channels.

HIGHER MIND: The highest vibration of the mind body, which knows truth and brings clarity to intuition and choice.

HIGHER SELF: The voice of the divine knowing; the personal manifestation of God Within.

JUDGMENT: The emotional theme that denies unity.

KARMA: The repetition of our experiential lessons of life until spiritual knowing is achieved, through the law of cause and effect.

KARMIC ATTACHMENTS: The attachment of energy to the emotional body from an overwhelming experience of life.

KUNDALINI: The fiery energy arising from the first chakra, which may spiral up the spinal cord, activating and balancing all the chakras of the body.

MIND BODY: A nonphysical subtle body that contains our intellectual, rational, logical thinking.

MULTIDIMENSIONAL NATURE: The concept of many co-existing and simultaneous dimensions of vibratory experience existing in concert and orchestrated by the Higher Self.

NADIS: The nonphysical pathways of ch'i from the chakras through the etheric body.

NEGATIVE SPACE/TIME: That realm that vibrates faster than the speed of light; the home of the subtle bodies.

PERNICIOUS EVIL: In Chinese medicine, this is an environmental factor that triggers disease; examples are wind, cold, fire, heat, dampness, dryness, and summer heat.

POSITIVE SPACE/TIME: That realm that vibrates at less than or equal to the speed of light; the home of the physical body.

PURE CONSCIOUSNESS: The impersonal, abstract aspect of God, experienced as unbounded, absolute, and infinite. The silence of Self, the "home" of all the laws of nature.

SEPARATION: The initial experience of taking form into duality; the companion of judgment.

SOLAR PLEXUS CHAKRA: The energy center located below the breastbone on the midline of the body. This chakra is the control center of the emotional body.

SPIRITUAL BODY: The highest vibratory nonphysical subtle body which connects all of our subtle bodies to the God-energy of life.

SUBTLE BODY: A general term for any nonphysical body that exists beyond normal third-dimension perception; specifically, the etheric, astral, mind, emotional, and spiritual bodies.

SYNCHRONICITY: A meaningful coincidence that connects an inner need with an outer event.

THIRD EYE: Located in the center of the forehead, this chakra is the connection to higher mind.

THOUGHTFORM: The manifestation of thought or emotion into matter or energy.

THROAT CHAKRA: The energy center that controls communication; it can be blocked or inhibited by the karma of judgment/separation.

UNITY CONSCIOUSNESS: When the inner Self and the outer Non-Self are merged together and perceived as one Self.

VIBRATIONAL MEDICINE: A holistic treatment that heals/balances multidimensionally, that is, both the physical body and the subtle bodies.

YIN/YANG: The polarity of creation. Yin represents the archetypal female energy; yang represents the archetypal male energy.

About the Author

Rick Phillips is a teacher and psychospiritual facilitator for the work of the Deva Foundation, of which he is one of the founders. He travels extensively, offering lectures and workshops on various themes of personal and planetary healing. In addition, he devotes much of his time to developing the charitable aspect of the Deva Foundation in its role of service and social action for the planet.

Rick lives with his wife, Paula, and his dog, Moishe, in the mountains near Santa Fe, New Mexico.

To contact Rick Phillips or to receive more information about the Deva Foundation, please contact:

Deva Foundation
Post Office Box 91
Glorieta, New Mexico 87535
USA
(505) 757-6752
FAX (505) 757-6752

or

Deva Foundation — Europe
Klingentalgraben 5
CH-4057 Basel
Switzerland
061-692-44-88

BOOKS OF RELATED INTEREST
BY BEAR & COMPANY

VIBRATIONAL MEDICINE
New Choices for Healing Ourselves
by Richard Gerber, M.D.

ECSTASY IS A NEW FREQUENCY
Teachings of The Light Institute
by Chris Griscom

EYE OF THE CENTAUR
A Visionary Guide into Past Lives
by Barbara Hand Clow

HEART OF THE CHRISTOS
Starseeding from the Pleiades
by Barbara Hand Clow

ORIGINAL BLESSING
A Primer in Creation Spirituality
by Matthew Fox

THE UNIVERSE IS A GREEN DRAGON
A Cosmic Creation Story
by Brian Swimme

DANCING WITH THE FIRE
Transforming Limitation Through Firewalking
by Michael Sky

Contact your local bookseller or write:
BEAR & COMPANY
P.O. Drawer 2860
Santa Fe, NM 87504